THE MANAGED CARE ANSWER BOOK

THE MANAGED CARE ANSWER BOOK

For Mental Health Professionals

by

Gayle McCracken Tuttle

and

Dianne Rush Woods

Routledge
Taylor & Francis Group
NEW YORK AND LONDON

First published 1997 by BRUNNER/MAZEL, INC.

This edition published 2014 by Routledge
605 Third Avenue, New York, NY 10017
2 Park Square, Milton Park, Abingdon, Oxon OX14 4RN

First issued in hardback 2017

Routledge is an imprint of the Taylor & Francis Group, an informa business

Library of Congress Cataloging-in-Publication Data

Tuttle, Gayle McCracken.
The managed care answer book for mental health professionals / by Gayle McCracken Tuttle and Dianne Rush Woods.
p. cm.
Includes bibliographical references.
ISBN 0-87630-848-5 (paper)
1. Managed mental health care. 2. Psychotherapy—Practice—United States. I. Woods, Dianne Rush. II. Title. III. Title: Managed care answer book.
[DNLM: 1. Managed Care Programs—examination questions. 2. Mental Health Services—examination questions. WM 18.2 T967m 1997]
RC465.6.T88 1997
362.2'0425—DC21
DNLM/DLC
for Library of Congress 97-13571
CIP

ISBN 13: 978-1-138-17912-7 (hbk)
ISBN 13: 978-0-87630-848-6 (pbk)

THE MANAGED CARE ANSWER BOOK

For Mental Health Professionals

by

Gayle McCracken Tuttle

and

Dianne Rush Woods

Routledge
Taylor & Francis Group
NEW YORK AND LONDON

First published 1997 by BRUNNER/MAZEL, INC.

This edition published 2014 by Routledge
605 Third Avenue, New York, NY 10017
2 Park Square, Milton Park, Abingdon, Oxon OX14 4RN

First issued in hardback 2017

Routledge is an imprint of the Taylor & Francis Group, an informa business

Library of Congress Cataloging-in-Publication Data

Tuttle, Gayle McCracken.
The managed care answer book for mental health professionals / by Gayle McCracken Tuttle and Dianne Rush Woods.
p. cm.
Includes bibliographical references.
ISBN 0-87630-848-5 (paper)
1. Managed mental health care. 2. Psychotherapy—Practice—United States. I. Woods, Dianne Rush. II. Title. III. Title: Managed care answer book.
[DNLM: 1. Managed Care Programs—examination questions. 2. Mental Health Services—examination questions. WM 18.2 T967m 1997]
RC465.6.T88 1997
362.2'0425—DC21
DNLM/DLC
for Library of Congress 97-13571
CIP

ISBN 13: 978-1-138-17912-7 (hbk)
ISBN 13: 978-0-87630-848-6 (pbk)

CONTENTS

FOREWORD

This book is intended as a resource and guide for all psychotherapists looking for answers to questions about the business of providing clinical services in a complex and rapidly changing marketplace. For nearly a decade—in our roles as a clinician and director of managed care provider relations, and as a journalist and speaker tracking industry trends and private practice issues—we have received hundreds of questions from psychotherapists across the country.

Each workshop and conference ends with hands still raised and frustrated psychotherapists walk away with unanswered questions about pressing business issues. What happens when I get dropped from a managed care panel? How do I get paid? Why can't I get on managed care panels? A common thread runs through the questions scribbled on slips of paper and the backs of business cards: Well into the industrialization of their profession, psychotherapists need nuts-and-bolts answers about the business of mental health treatment.

The Managed Care Answer Book is an extended Q&A session where issues are tackled from a provider's perspective.

Questions and answers about the business side of mental health care are divided into chapters that address the various phases and facets of managed care. Clinicians should skip from one to the next as they move through stages of practice and market development. Readers steering away from third-party payments will find ideas for new private-pay products, while group practices may be more interested in pricing formulas and contracting issues.

This collection of resources, examples, and explanations was created to help clinicians understand and anticipate market changes, and to find a place within the new delivery system where they can practice effectively and profitably.

GAYLE MCCRACKEN TUTTLE
DIANNE RUSH WOODS

1

Psychotherapy: Cottage to Industry

Look to your left, look to your right; one of you won't be here next year.

Alan Savitz, M.D., President, PacifiCare Behavioral Health

The decision by employers to hire managed care firms to control the delivery of mental health services under insurance benefit plans has probably had more impact on your practice than any other single factor. Still, there are clinicians who dismiss the mention of managed behavioral health care as something that happens to someone else.

Psychotherapy took roots as a cottage industry beginning in the 1950s as business and industry offered richer insurance coverage to compete for skilled employees. Legislative mandates fed the idea of behavioral health care as a guaranteed benefit, and psychotherapy as a profession enjoyed the results.

Then came the wake-up call of the last decade: Mental health providers are not immune to economic forces. Corporate belt-tightening, downsizings, layoffs, outsourcing—all buzzwords of the 1990s marketplace—have been added to the glossaries of psychotherapists in business suits. Managed care has evolved as a system of cost-containment, research-based treatment plans, and setting standards for services and payment.

Acknowledging those changes and the resulting impact on local market systems is a critical first step to survival in private practice. Some group practice owners say they have to evaluate their business plans, structures and marketing goals and consider revisions every six months. Managed care mergers and acquisitions, the dissolution of indemnity insurance markets and privatization of public sector programs all threaten the private practitioner.

Tracking national trends is a start. Knowing the current local market, anticipating how soon, and to what extent those national trends will impact your ability to sell clinical services are the real issues. Managed behavioral care firms are being acquired by venture capitalists, insurance companies and pharmaceutical firms, moving decision making on mental health and substance abuse matters from clinical directors to business and financial specialists.

Fee-for-service payments will be the exception to the managed care rule, eliminating the idea of $60, $70, $90, or $150 for an hour of therapy. The therapy hour as we know it is going to be very different. Under capitation plans, providers will be paid for treating a case, or with a set dollar amount per member, per month. Managed care plans for public and private sector clients will include new fee schedules to reflect where treatment is delivered, intensity of services, and session times beginning with 15-minute consultation.

Private practitioners will compete by lowering their fees, or by adding value to their services. Value will be defined as access through extended hours; services delivered in homes, nursing centers, hospital emergency rooms, doctor's offices; or wellness and preventive services. Providers who have adapted to lower fees under managed care will be more willing to negotiate fees and payment plans in order to compete for a growing out-of-pocket clientele.

In some cases, individual providers will work under retainers, receiving $1,000 to $5,000 each month to see clients from a particular company. Providers in a variety of group structures and sizes will work as part of integrated delivery systems connecting them to hospitals, day treatment programs, insurances companies, and Health Maintenance Organizations (HMOs).

There will be fewer providers. The lucrative markets of the '60s, '70s and '80s will have disappeared. Group practices will capture large amounts of business based on their efficiency and economies of scale. Regional hospital systems, physician-owned practices and large behavioral health care groups will have an excellent opportunity to dominate local markets through direct contracts with employers. Some national managed behavioral health care firms will view those new alliances as customers for their provider network and utilization management services, turning the tables again on client and customer relationships. Consider these trends in terms of your community, its employers, your existing client base, and how you want to practice tomorrow. (See Exhibit 1.1.)

BASICS

Q What are clinician concerns about managed care?

A The concerns that we hear voiced most often are that managed care compromises client well-being and threatens confidentiality. Therapists complain about lower fees (Horowitz & Pollack, 1993) and find it difficult to manage communications with clients and managed care firms. Increased paperwork and the expense of keeping pace with technology have driven many therapists from the field. Concerns about confidentiality and materials released to managed care reviewers have made providers uneasy. Many who remain in private practice are shifting to a business orientation, where therapy is viewed as a marketable product. Cost is weighed against value, to arrive at quality—usually redefined as levels of patient functionality.

Q When I listen to managed care talk, I start to buy into it. Then I think about myself as the patient and I know it isn't right. What can I do?

A Many solo providers and those in group practices believe that the quality of their clinical care has improved under managed care, and that more patients have access to at least some care. When managed care is defined as the measurement of therapy results according to standards set by clinicians, many therapists say they are more confident about their services. When it is defined as a payment system with treatment decisions made outside of the clinical setting, therapists feel very compromised.

For those who choose to accept third-party payment for services, some form of care management, utilization review, quality assurance, and outcomes measurement is a given. Provider involvement in defining quality of care and treatment standards is critical to an effective system. Data from actual practice patterns and provider profiles are being used to shape, train, and redirect providers within behavioral health care systems. Micromanagement and outside utilization review are being phased out.

EXHIBIT 1.1. Trends to Track.

1. **Backward integration is on the way**. Expect an increase in HMO coverage of mental health/chemical dependency treatment. National and regional HMOs are developing their own behavioral health panels, in many cases integrating their services with staff model primary-care physician practices. Practitioners should apply to HMOs, as well as to managed behavioral health "carve-out" firms—those specializing in mental health management.

2. **Indemnity insurers will go managed care.** It started with the pooling of 23 million lives when insurance company Aetna, Inc. merged with U.S. Healthcare, a large HMO. Another example is Prudential, Inc.'s decision to form a joint venture with Value Behavioral Health and Merit Behavioral Care Corporation—two of the largest carve-out mental health firms—to serve its clients. Indemnity health insurance premiums are falling as employees choose HMOs and states contract with managed care firms to cover Medicaid and uninsured populations. More large insurance firms will purchase managed care networks, establish their own provider panels, or form joint ventures with managed care firms.

3. **Provider-managed care will dominate** in many regional markets, as physicians and behavioral health care providers join forces, or develop separate systems designed to eliminate third-party payers. Their target markets will be hospital-driven systems and employers.

4. **The carve-out industry is in a great deal of turmoil.** The mental health industry giants have essentially trained behavioral health provider groups to do their job of utilization review, case management, outcomes measurement, and quality review. There is a great deal of opportunity for sophistocated provider groups to go directly to middle-sized employers (100-plus employees) and sell a managed mental health product, bypassing the mental health firms.

5. **Providers will comply with treatment standards** as they join managed care firms in seeking accreditation by national quality monitors. Large quality-conscious employers are embracing national accreditation standards under the National Committee for Quality Assurance (NCQA) and the Joint Commission on Accreditation for Healthcare Organizations (JCAHO). Stringent criteria that include site visits and record reviews for network providers have been extended to behavioral health care.

6. Network provider panels will be smaller. Expect a 20% decrease in network size. The average specialty managed care firm panel is about 30,000. It's too big and too unwieldy to manage. Managed care firms spend about $100 per provider per year for primary-source verification. The entire credentialing process can cost $300 to $400 for each provider. That's why managed care firms discourage new applications unless there is a need for service. New NCQA standards defining subscriber access may force expansion in some areas.

7. Sophisticated group practices will be closer partners with managed care firms. As utilization management companies shift clinical and administrative responsibilities to those groups, they will wield greater local market control. Solo providers should market to those groups, as well as to companies, employers, hospital systems, and private-pay clients.

8. More providers will look for markets outside of managed care. Expect a resurgence of aggressive provider marketing to private-pay clients. Clinicians will cut their fees, work smarter and cheaper, and manage their own quality and outcomes to lure dissatisfied clients away from managed care systems.

9. Proving value and showing savings in medical costs will be paramount for provider professional associations, as they push for parity. Employers still see mental health benefits as a costly add-on. Now is the time for providers to think multidisciplinary, multispecialty, and to use cost-offset studies to show employers value in reduced sick days, lower medical costs, and more productive workers.

10. New pricing structures, including case rates and capitation, will prevail. While ethical concerns and patient complaints have pushed one regional HMO to return to fees-for-service, the general trend is toward at-risk contracting. Provider-managed delivery systems, however, tend to hold the risk within the business structure and do not pass it along to contracted network providers. Managed care will drop reduced fee rates to encourage providers to take risk pricing.

11. Specialty services will be the key to new markets. For example there are never enough child psychiatrists.

Other providers are choosing to opt out of the third-party payment system and are slashing their fees by up to 50% in order to recapture an out-of-pocket clientele.

(For the stages of managed behavioral health care, see Exhibit 1.2.)

Q What is the definition of managed care?

A During the early generations of managed behavioral health care, it was often defined as the payment for treatment by anyone other than the patient, and centered on companies hired to manage the cost of delivering that treatment by limiting access. As mentioned earlier, that definition is being broadened through consumer awareness and provider participation. We think this description by Shore and Beigle (1996) is one of clearest definitions of the emerging system:

> Managed mental health care companies and mental health care providers must work together to develop new methods of practice that meet the particular challenges posed by managed care. These challenges affect medical ethics, the definition of mental illnesses, the management of limited resources, and accountability of providers. Managed care defines and treats mental illness in terms of the ability of a person to function, while traditional mental health care is concerned with long-term treatment of underlying illnesses. Mental health care is becoming geared towards the needs of larger populations rather than those of individual patients in one-on-one meetings. Managed care is also causing psychiatrists to see more severely ill patients. Fees tend to be based on the complexity of illness rather than on the training of the provider. Finally, managed care permits case managers, sometimes with less training than the provider, to evaluate the quality of care. This arrangement may be replaced by large provider groups that assume financial risk and manage their own care.

Q Can managed care providers say to a patient: "We will give you only eight sessions. We will not pretend you will be cured. You will have to pay for the rest on your own"?

A That's exactly what managed care is about. Benefit plans are built around definitions of medical necessity, diagnostic codes, and measurements of the patient's ability to function. The goal for employers and managed care firms is to return patients to a functional level on the job, in school, and as part of their families. Once the goals of a treatment plan, based on medical necessity, have been met, managed care firms are slow to authorize additional sessions. The key for providers is to diagnose carefully and to include case managers in setting realistic goals in treatment plans that comply with the patient's benefit plan.

EXHIBIT 1.2. Stages of Managed Behavioral Health Care.

First Generation: Restricted Access
- Utilization review
- Large copayments
- Retroactive claims denial

Second Generation: Managed Benefit Utilization
- Provider selection, credentialing
- Managed care friendly providers
- Bull's-eye panel selection, referrals

Third generation: Managing the Care
- Managed networks
- Continuum of care
- Provider training

Fourth generation: Managed Outcomes
- Provider/patient profiling
- Preventive services
- Home-based services
- Backward integration (HMOs)
- Primary care emphasis

Fifth Generation: Provider-Managed Care
- Provider-sponsored networks
- Disease management
- Consumer responsive
- Accreditation
- Managed care organization (MCO) joint ventures

Q How can I predict how soon managed care will affect my practice?

A Your own client files may be the best indicator. Who are your clients insured by now, and has their coverage changed in the last year? Has your client base dropped? Are your colleagues signing more managed care contracts? Read local business journals and the business sections of local newspapers to learn about employer choices of managed care companies. Ask the state insurance commissioner for a listing of licensed HMOs and Preferred Provider Organizations (PPOs), and for those with license applications pending.

Q How many managed mental health care companies are there?

A The number rose as high as 400 during the early 1980s, but has dropped considerably through industry mergers and acquisitions. Now, fewer than two dozen large national managed behavioral health care firms control nearly 90% of lives under plans with mental health benefits. OPEN MINDS reports in its 1995 industry survey that 111 million Americans, or 50% of the insured population, are covered by some form of managed behavioral health care plan. That does not take into account, however, HMOs with behavioral health networks, regional and statewide managed behavioral health care firms, and companies specializing in partial hospitalization or day treatment, or that own or manage behavioral group practices. There were 562 HMO plans and 763 PPO plans operating in 1993 and 90% of those offered psychiatric benefits (*Managed Care Digest,* 1996). The larger mental health carve-out firms are listed in Appendix C.

Q As providers, we feel we're being micromanaged to death. We have to call managed care companies after two or five sessions and beg for more. Will this end?

A Yes, but not without a price. Managed care firms are sick of micromanagement, too. They are eager to shift the task to providers, along with the responsibility and the cost. That's why you're seeing the move toward smaller panels and stronger relationships with select group practices.

The trend among industry leaders is to pinpoint providers of quality, efficient care for volume referrals. Those providers will be spared intrusive reviews, and will receive approval for 10 to 15 sessions—if the managed care firm has seen a pattern of that provider completing treatment in fewer than 15 sessions (Garfield & Bergin, 1986). The provider is responsible, however, for documenting interventions and results—in effect, creating new benchmarks.

Another option that is taking hold with many managed care firms involves redesigning the benefits structure to allow sessions up to the average actually provided for a certain diagnosis. One benchmark in these systems is that treatment is most effective at 13 to 14 sessions, with a diminishing rate of return beyond that number (Garfield & Bergin, 1986). Utilization review would be reserved for inpatient, day treatment, and partial hospitalization.

Q What is meant by shifting paradigms?

A Shifting paradigms has become an industry buzz phrase for changing treatment models and theories to fit a market that is driven by employer needs and budget constraints. For clinicians, that means a shift to brief therapy models, treating patients according to care standards accepted by managed care firms, and measuring and reporting the results of their care.

Q Who will hold the managed care firms accountable? Will it be the government or mental health professionals?

A Government oversight will be limited to contracts with managed care firms for public sector clients, including Medicare and those under Medicaid waivers managed by states. Additionally, the Department of Justice can be expected to monitor managed care firms, as well as large group practices, that are operating under capitation and case rate contracts and present the risk of underutilization.

Increasingly, large employers are demanding both cost and quality accountability from managed care firms. In turn, outside credentialing agencies, including the National Committee on Quality Assurance (NCQA) and the Joint Commission on Accreditation of Healthcare Organizations (JCAHO), have set standards of care for HMOs and PPOs. The NCQA has proposed operating standards specific to behavioral health care firms. The managed care firms are also attempting to monitor themselves through the American Managed Behavioral Healthcare Association (AMBHA).

Q Although HMOs claim that confidentiality exists, a former patient told me that he was quoted higher rates when he applied for more life insurance because he had been treated for depression. Can HMOs guarantee confidentiality?

A HMOs can guarantee as much confidentiality as anyone else. They are bound by the same laws that providers are bound by in that they must keep records separate and they must get signatures to release information. But some of them report to a large database, giving numerical codes for all of their clients. There is a possibility that insurance companies access this database to determine how to rate policies. The Work Group for the Computer-Based Behavioral Health and Human Services Record, made up of providers and professional association representatives, has recommended a number of steps to tighten database security, including card, hand, or fingerprint scanning of those with access to records; encryption of data; and audit trail tracking (Webman, 1994). Managed care firms already use passwords and access codes.

The only way anyone can ensure confidentiality is to be treated under another name and pay cash. Key reasons are that providers are mandated to share material with the courts and protective services where there is a question of abuse or intent to harm another person. Providers cannot guarantee absolute confidentiality, and neither can HMOs.

The provider can refuse to release information to the managed care firm, but unless the company has information that allows it to determine medical necessity, the treatment won't be covered. The fact that payment will not be made based on limited information makes it important for the clinician to discuss with the client the impact of a decision not to release information to a third-party payer.

Q In Minnesota, large business buying groups have indicated their desire to contract directly with provider groups. Do you see this as a stronger trend for the future?

A Absolutely. As specialty managed care firms have implemented cost-cutting measures, they have passed on to providers many responsibilities for quality, utilization review, and outcomes measurement. Those providers (usually structured group practices) have learned the role of the managed care firm. Now, employers are beginning to ask: Why do we need a managed care firm? This opens the door to providers who are prepared to negotiate directly with employers to manage and deliver mental health and substance abuse treatment. The opportunities are especially attractive for group practices that can contract with hospital delivery systems and regional employers.

Q **What are some of the factors working against the large managed care companies?**

A Such factors include the following:

1. The initial savings produced by limiting access to providers and services were viewed favorably by employers, but the companies have not been able to produce significant additional savings. Ironically, early cost-cutting successes have worked against the long-term stability of carve-out firms.
2. An 800 number or the long-distance management of most large managed care firms creates a carpetbagger image in regional markets. The companies often don't understand, or they overlook, regional differences in economic and employer needs.
3. Managed care carve-outs no longer are perceived as innovators of cutting-edge technology and health care management, but as fat cats who are skimming the cream from the top of the health care dollar.
4. Small regional managed care firms gobbled up in industry mergers have lost their identities. Many employers believe that their industry focus has shifted from service to profit.

Q **What about the impact of managed care on Medicaid service for children, adolescents, and their families?**

A The poor and uninsured are going to share the advantages and disadvantages of managed mental health care that insured employees and their dependents have been adjusting to for the last 10 to 15 years. At least 34 states have Medicaid waivers in place as of this writing, and all are considering some sort of federal waiver that would allow state governments to contract with private managed care firms for behavioral, substance abuse, and various other services.

The states, eager to save money, are pushing to privatize as many programs as possible in one sweep—in many cases, adding foster care, forensic patients, and child welfare to the behavioral health deals. There are serious questions about how well managed care firms will be able to handle public populations with more severe illnesses than have been managed under employer plans.

Since the mandate is to lower costs, managed care firms will be offering less restricted levels of treatment to public-sector clients. Managed care doesn't always mean that the people won't get care, but that care will often be delivered through partial programs, day treatment centers, therapy groups, and community resources rather than inpatient programs. In fact, access is likely to be somewhat broader for the public population. In-home care will be a much bigger piece of the managed public-sector program because of compliance issues that would force higher costs for more intensive treatment if patients don't take medications and follow treatment plans.

For managed care firms, it means recruiting a new network of providers experienced in crisis intervention, the treatment of serious disorders, and working with minority and poor populations. Often a regional alliance of community mental health centers will be the hub of those networks. Capitated programs under Medicaid waivers are running from $17 to $30 per covered life, which is much higher than the usual $3.50 per member, per month, under employer plans.

DOLLARS AND CENTS

Q Must economic/business success determine quality of care?

A The quality of clinical service delivery is ethically and legally the responsibility of the clinician. Managed care companies determine whether the length of stay in treatment desired by the clinician and client meet the clinical criteria established by the company and whether they will pay for services. The clinicians must decide how services are delivered according to what is authorized under the client's benefits package and the client's understanding of his or her needs. This includes explaining thoroughly the nature of the contract with the managed care firm. For example: "Your company typically authorizes up to 10 sessions. During the first session, I will be assessing the clinical situation by listening to what you say and asking a series of questions. I will report some information to the managed care company and it will authorize sessions. If I feel that you need more than 10 sessions and the company refuses to authorize additional sessions, then you and I can talk about continuing treatment, at your expense, at the rate your managed care company currently pays me."

Managed care firms determine whether you are paid for additional sessions. Your fee schedule and the expectations that you set in the initial session determine whether you will be able to continue treatment, if you feel it is necessary, once the authorized sessions are completed. Some clients won't be able to pay for additional sessions. If additional care is needed, you should refer the client to a community resource and document the referral in the chart.

Q Do employers really care about quality and accreditation? Isn't price still the bottom line?

A Large national employers understand accreditation and quality assurance, and are requiring compliance. But small to middle-size employers are still buying price. And most still see behavioral health benefits as pricey add-ons with no proof of savings on the medical side. "Business people by and large believe that most people seeking mental health treatment are the worried well, or are very, very sick," says Alan Savitz, M.D., president of PacifiCare Behavioral Health. "They see it as a black hole."

Employer concern for quality will vary with location and market penetration. Once HMO growth picks up, expect closer attention to quality issues. Competition among specialty managed mental health firms, and between those companies and insurers, is forcing premiums down. In order to be competitive, managed care firms are shifting administrative tasks to providers, whose costs are rising. How those economics play out, and the degree of success that provider associations have in convincing employers of the value of their services, will determine what employers will pay for in the future. If pressed too hard, some employers will choose to provide only those services that protect them from liability risks. Leo H. Bradman, a psychologist and the head of Bradman/UniPsych Cos., a large Florida provider network that contracts directly with employers, summarizes the employer's bottom line as "little noise and no problems." Employers are most concerned about complying with the Americans with Disabilities Act, the Department of Transportation drug-testing rules, and with cutting Workers' Compensation costs. Those are clues for providers to use in developing employer consultation, supervisor training, and risk management products (Yandrick, 1995).

Q Since managed care companies are profit oriented and are paid by employers whether or not they cover services provided, is there not a conflict of interest?

A Managed care firms earn higher profits by delivering medically necessary services at the least restrictive level of care. Managed care firms have never tried to hide the fact that they exist as businesses and, as such, have a goal of making money. Most, however, were formed with the intention of delivering quality care. It is important to remember that the companies exist because employers hire them to contain the costs of benefits delivery. The question of conflict of interest is being faced not only by managed care firms, but also by providers who deliver services under capitated contracts. As an investor in a delivery system, will the provider first protect his or her pocketbook or the interests of the client? A Department of Justice task force is considering new guidelines that would extend to group practices to guard against underutilization of services in capitated plans. That's a reversal of antifraud measures under indemnity plans designed to discourage overutilization of services.

Q Is managed care actually saving employers money?

A Yes. Competition among health care providers and increasing HMO participation have been credited with holding down health care costs for employers in 1995 and limiting projected increases for 1996 to 3% or less. The average cost increase in health care coverage per employee in 1995 was $3,653, up only slightly from $3,644 in 1994, according to a national survey of 2,764 public and private employers by A. Foster Higgins (1996). Similarly, a study by Towers Perrin (1996) projects flat costs for HMO coverage in 1996, with non-HMO plans expected to increase by 4%, or double 1995's 2% increase.

Q Will managed care cost more in the long run because of repeats of brief therapy?

A Most managed care firms support the Harvard Community Mental Health Plan model of intermittent recycled therapy. The idea is that people will come in for short periods to work on presenting problems, and then return later to work on new problems. That model predicts a long-term savings from reduced inpatient costs, rather than from reducing outpatient psychotherapy.

A study of a California public utility working with a managed care firm showed a complete reversal from 70% inpatient treatment to 70% outpatient treatment, with more employees accessing care after two years under the managed care plan. Even with increased utilization at $60 or $70 per session, the costs were lower than inpatient days at $500 to $700.

A number of studies indicate that both private-practice patients and patients of community mental health centers expect therapy to last between five and eight sessions (Garfield & Bergin, 1986), precisely the outpatient benchmark arrived at by both managed care firms and provider-run managed care group practices.

Q Are any good studies available that show that behavioral health care cuts medical costs?

A There are a number of good studies supporting cost offset. "The Cost of Addictive and Mental Disorders and Effectiveness of Treatment," released by the Substance Abuse and Mental Health Services Administration (SAMHSA), documents health care cost decreases of up to 55% following treatment for alcoholism. It also shows a decrease from $263 spent per month by a family with a member suffering from a mental disorder to $208 per month after one year of treatment, and to $162 per month after two years of behavioral health treatment. Copies of the report are issued free by writing to the Data Analysis Center, SAMHSA, 5600 Fishers Lane, Room 12105, Rockville, MD 20857.

Q Have efforts been made to control the administrative cost of managed care firms, particularly the absurdly high salaries of managed care executives?

A Efforts are in place, both internally and externally, to control the cost of managed care companies. Brokerage firms, such as Anderson, Anderson & Mercer, advise employers on how much they should pay for services and try to make sure they are guaranteed the best prices possible. Managed care firms were built by investors with a goal of making profits. Executives have been rewarded financially for reducing health care costs. There has been considerable public backlash in response to the hundreds of thousands of dollars in salaries and dividends going to a handful of top executives. Several have made public gestures by refusing raises and cutting their own salaries.

The average salary for male managed care executives reached $94,731 in 1995 and $64,224 for female executives that same year, according to a national industry survey (*"The Managed Care Executive,"* 1996). The survey reported a 1995 average salary range of $26,000 to $195,000 for managed care professional employees, with average raises of 10.57%.

Salaries and bonuses contingent on meeting sales goals, holding customers, and decreasing costs are likely to remain high. But mental health carve-out firms are operating on narrow profit margins and are cutting other costs internally by reducing staff, shifting responsibilities to provider group practices, and utilizing computer systems.

Q What are medical savings accounts? How do they work?

A Employers buy coverage with high deductibles and put the money they would have spent on premiums for insurance with lower deductibles into flexible spending accounts for employees. Employees turn in receipts for medical care, child care, elder care, or other work-life expenses to be reimbursed by the employer from the accounts. The accounts are usually maintained at about $5,000. If the employee doesn't turn in receipts, he or she loses the money. Medical savings accounts (MSA) are intended to supplement, not replace, major medical coverage.

Q Where does mental health fit into this picture?

A There are still many employers who see behavioral health care as an expensive add-on. Pushing behavioral health care out of the managed benefit pool and into an optional spending area would allow employees more freedom in choosing providers and services. Some mental health providers view medical savings accounts, or flexible spending accounts, as a positive way to encourage private-pay clients. Other providers see them as a threat to mental health services, thinking that employers may consider the flexible spending option a substitute for mental health benefits.

PROVIDER ISSUES

Q What is meant by bull's-eye panel selection?

A Managed care companies have tiered their provider panels, moving the select providers and group practices to the center of an imaginary bull's-eye target. (See Exhibit 1.3.) Those providers in the center receive high volumes of referrals because the companies know they will adhere to practice patterns that meet their treatment guidelines. They have implemented quality assurance systems, follow managed care practice standards, and are staffed to triage, assess, and refer patients quickly. In general, providers on the outer rim of the "bull's-eye" are individual practitioners who see few managed care patients.

EXHIBIT 1.3. Bull's eye panel selection.

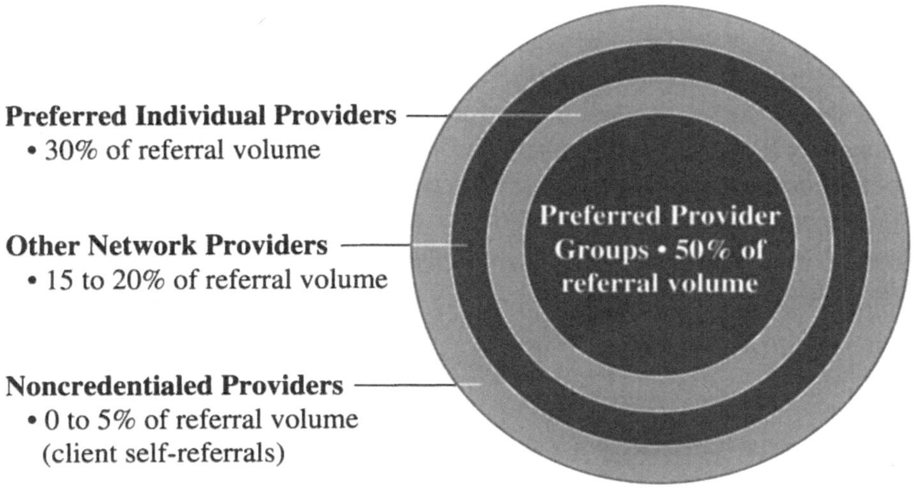

Q As someone who is involved in training psychology and family therapy interns, I am concerned about the effect of managed care on training programs. What influence will managed care have on training? Can we afford to continue training?

A During the first generations of managed behavioral health care, the carve-out firms and HMOs rarely allowed interns and residents to treat patients under their plans. There is discussion now among managed care firms and professional associations about reversing that policy. Part of the problem is that training organizations have to adjust their fees upward by between 10% and 25% to cover supervisor fees. While managed care firms have been reluctant to pay the additional fees, some are considering contracts with university clinical training programs.

Q In the view of managed care companies, how well prepared are master's level clinicians to treat complicated diagnoses? How do we convince managed care companies of our abilities to treat severe mental illnesses?

A Based on levels of severity under standard diagnoses as established in the latest (fourth) edition of the *Diagnostic and Statistical Manual of Mental Disorders* (DSM-IV), up to 60% of cases are routinely referred to master's level clinicians. When there is major depression or other complicating issues, the concept of one-stop shopping becomes very attractive to managed care firms. This is where multispecialty group practices that include a psychiatrist and medication management fare well. There are cases, however, where the client is referred to a master's-level clinician or a psychologist for case management and therapy, but an outside psychiatrist handles psychotropic medications. While the second model often works nicely, master's-level clinicians enhance their market position by aligning themselves with multispecialty groups.

Q Some managed care arrangements do not support marital therapy as medically necessary. Do you have any suggestions as to how to advocate for better benefits?

A Most managed care firms actually support coverage of marital therapy, recognizing the cost-offset value of early preventive care. Few, however, have been able to convince employers that not providing marital therapy can result in more expensive treatment for both marriage partners for anxiety, depression, or other disorders.

It is important to note the role of the national professional organizations in the relationship with managed care companies. The National Federation of Societies for Clinical Social Work, the American Association for Marriage and Family Therapy, the National Association of Social Workers, the American Psychological Association, and the American Psychiatric Association all oppose medical necessity as a barrier to payment for V-code therapy.

Working through state chapters of national associations to deliver to employers a message that marital therapy is cost-effective is the starting point for advocacy work.

Q Many managed care firms in my state won't allow me to be one of their practitioners. Should this be illegal? What can we do about this restriction of trade?

A Managed care firms are able to control costs by referring to providers who have agreed to accept reduced fees and to practice within the company's treatment guidelines. Those firms argue that they can't achieve cost savings or control the quality of care if they are not able to choose their network providers. In order to be accredited, managed care firms must credential every provider, with primary-source verification of education, licensing, malpractice coverage, or malpractice actions. Managed care firms have estimated that building a credentialing file on a single provider can take several hours and cost $300 to $400.

Providers in many states have turned to any-willing-provider (AWP) laws in the hope of forcing managed care firms to accept all qualified clinicians who agree to a company's policies and payment terms. By 1996, 24 states had 28 any-willing-provider laws on the books. Most were passed between 1983 and 1994. In 1995, of 79 such bills considered, only three were passed (*The 1995 State*, 1995). While these laws can compel a managed care firm to include a provider on a network panel, they do not require the firm to make referrals to that provider.

Managed care firms rate providers on the basis of volume within geographic areas. This goes back to the bull's-eye panel and tiering of preferred providers to receive high volumes of referrals. The "A" providers are those providers whom the managed care company wanted and solicited, and the

"B" providers are those whom the managed care company has been forced to include. Providers in some states are abandoning AWP battles in favor of "right-to-know" and "point-of-service" measures. The new measures are a mixed bag, calling for subscribers to be able to select providers at the time service is delivered, to set penalties for managed care firms that don't explain in writing why a provider is rejected or dropped from a panel, to instruct companies to disclose to subscribers information about financial incentives to providers who limit treatment, and, in some cases, to ban "gag" clauses.

Another issue for providers is state licensure. There are still a number of states that do not license certain providers, whereas most managed care firms will only accept licensed providers. That becomes less of an issue as group practices and delivery systems move to capitated pricing arrangements where the system or group decides who will deliver care, within the constraints of the employer's benefit design.

Q Will the discrimination in the mental health field end? Physicians can join panels if they agree to terms. Mental health providers are being told they cannot join.

A Inclusion in a network is based on the need of the managed care organization to provide a panel for clients in that area. Panels usually have a ratio, something like 1:1,000 per population in the area. If there are many providers in the area, then the managed care company has no need to recruit additional therapists. It's a case of supply and demand. If the demand for therapists' services increases in the area, then the managed care firm will recruit more providers, usually offering specialized services to complement its core groups. If the firms lose contracts, or employers reduce benefit packages, the network is likely to be reduced. Additionally, managed care firms are working more with structured group practices that are willing to share risks for patient care and costs. In some cases, network providers may receive as few as one to three new referrals per contract each year, whereas select group practices can receive up to 70% of a company's referrals. That calls into question the need for any-willing-provider legislation that can force a company to include a therapist on a panel. However, managed care firms do not feel an obligation to guarantee referrals for all providers in a region. Nearly 25,000 new psychotherapists are licensed each year. They are added to 300,000 already practicing. Based on the 1:1,000 ratio, HMOs estimate that they need about one third of those licensed mental health providers.

Q After we follow your recommendations, when do we make a living?

A The field is changing rapidly, so the answer to that question doesn't guarantee a "living," but rather addresses the revolutionary times in which we live. Prudent business structuring, effective contracting, niche marketing, and greater cost awareness are factors that will support an individual's livelihood. It is important to note that no field of practice is guaranteed survival. The "psychebusiness" experienced unprecedented growth during the 1960s, 1970s and 1980s. We are now undergoing the purposeful downsizing of a business that is part of industrialization. Therapists are going out of business, accepting lower or flattened incomes, working part-time for agencies, or becoming employees of managed care systems. This is part of a political and social climate in which all forms of service delivery are subject to cynicism and to questions as to whether the service is needed, and if so, how it can be delivered more efficiently.

REFERENCES

A. Foster Higgins & Co., Inc. (1996, Jan. 30). *National survey of employer-sponsored health plans 1995.* New York: Author.

American Psychiatric Association. (1994). *Diagnostic and Statistical Manual of Mental Disorders* (Fourth Edition) (DSM-IV) Washington, DC: APA.

Garfield, S., & Bergin, A. (1986). Research on client variables in psychotherapy (pp. 190–228). *Handbook of psychotherapy and behavior change, Third Edition,* New York: Wiley.

Hymowitz, C., & Pollack, E. (1995, July 13). Psychobattle: Cost-cutting firms monitor couch time. Sensing a loss of control, doctors call it quits. *Wall Street Journal,* p. A-1.

Managed Care Digest (1994). HMO and PPO editions. Kansas City, MO: Marion Merrell Dow.

Oss, M. (1995, Apr.) *Trends in behavioral health financing.* Gettysburg, PA: OPEN MINDS.

Shore, M., & Beigle, A. (1996). Synopsis of the challenges posed by managed care. *The New England Journal of Medicine, 334*(2), 116–119.

The managed care executive's salary and benefits survey (1996). Wall Township NJ: Managed Care Information Center.

The 1995 state managed care legislative resource (1995). Washington DC: American Managed Care and Review Association.

Towers Perrin (1996, Jan.). *Towers Perrin health cost benchmarking study.* New York: Author.

Webman, D. (1994). Provider recommendations for safeguarding patient confidentiality. *Behavioral Healthcare Tomorrow, 3*(1), 33, 37–38.

Yandrick, R. (1995). Behavioral risk management: The preventive approach to reducing workplace problems. *Behavioral Healthcare Tomorrow, 4*(5), 31–35.

2

How It Works: For You, or Against You

Providers just can't do things and bill anymore. Services must be provided within the context of organized systems of care using a full continuum of care with clinical and fiscal accountability through documented and measurable outcomes.

Mary Jane England, Past President, American Psychiatric Association

Psychotherapists treating patients who are covered by any sort of third-party payment plan will work under a managed care system. There are options: reject insurance, Medicaid, and CHAMPUS (the federal health plan for military enrollees, retirees and their dependents) payments; sell services to private-pay patients; take a job; or change careers. For providers who want to remain in private practice, the optimal choice will be to diversify service offerings, become more business-minded, and sell to a mixed market of managed care, community programs, out-of-pocket clients, employers, and contracting agencies.

That relieves some of the pressure for providers to acquiesce to every managed care firm's demands. Providers who achieve a strong practice balance will be able to select the managed care firms they work with, based on volume of referrals and similar treatment philosophies.

Providers who have chosen to work with managed care have gone through a developmental stage, starting with denial and resistance, and moving through retraining and product development to teamwork. (See Exhibit 2.1.) Some have used responses to managed care firm questions about practice patterns as a way to reconcile their own clinical issues with industry demands. A good example is a treatment philosophy developed by Maurie Cullen, a California social worker. (See Exhibit 2.2.)

This chapter answers the basic questions that arise for providers working with one or 20 managed care firms, and for those providers seeking to create their own systems for managing care and measuring effectiveness.

THE RATING GAME

Q I keep hearing about being a team player with managed care. Who is on the team besides me and the patient?

EXHIBIT 2.1. Development Stages of Managed Care Providers.

NEW MARKET
Denial
Minimize How It Affects Me
How Good Things Were
It Won't Happen to Me
Shock/Numbness
Everything-as-Usual Attitude

EMERGING MARKET
Commitment/Involvement
Moving Ahead
Focusing on Direction
Teamwork
Cooperation

YOUNG MARKET
Resistance
Anger
Loss and Hurt
Stubbornness
Blaming
Complaining

ESTABLISHED MARKET
Exploration/Adaptation
Seeing Possibilities
Clarifying Goals
Exploring Alternatives
Indecisiveness
Learning New Skills
Creativity

Source: Tamara Cagney, Pleasanton, CA. Reprinted with permission.

EXHIBIT 2.2. Treatment Philosophy.

Believing in the worth and dignity of each person who enters my practice, my therapeutic approach with clients encompasses several key factors. The first task in the therapeutic process is to provide an atmosphere of safety, receptivity and trust. Clients need a safe environment in which they may speak openly about their concerns and fears. I recognize the difficulty clients have in confiding in a stranger and the courage that it takes for them to begin psychotherapy.

Secondly, I employ an approach that is a synthesis of psychodynamic theory, ego psychology, self psychology, family and community systems and, when appropriate, 12-step involvement. As a clinical social worker, I am aware of the necessity of completing a thorough bio-psycho-social assessment. This means exploring the family history as it relates to family illnesses, including alcoholism and other forms of compulsive disorders. I have extensive experience in chemical dependency assessment and understand the importance of not colluding in the denial associated with this insidious disease. I also recognize the impact of chemical dependency on those who indirectly suffer from substance abuse: the family members, parents, spouses and children. Also, when appropriate, clients are referred to various community resources to assist them with 12-step recovery, vocation assistance, medical evaluations, academic planning, and other specific needs.

Rather than view clients as "diseases" or "cases," I focus on the most effective means of mobilizing a client's strengths. I do not believe in creating undue dependence on psychotherapy and will help a client to resolve the conflict that brought them in for help and guide them through termination as they develop their strengths and abilities. The door is left open for them to reenter therapy, if at some later point, further help is needed.

A The team in an integrated delivery system model can include the behavioral health provider, the primary care doctor, the managed care firm, the employer, the third-party administrator of a self-funded plan or the insurer, the home health agency, the patient, the family, and public support systems, in-cluding child welfare, the courts, and community resources. (See Exhibit 2.3.)

EXHIBIT 2.3. The Managed Care Treatment Team.

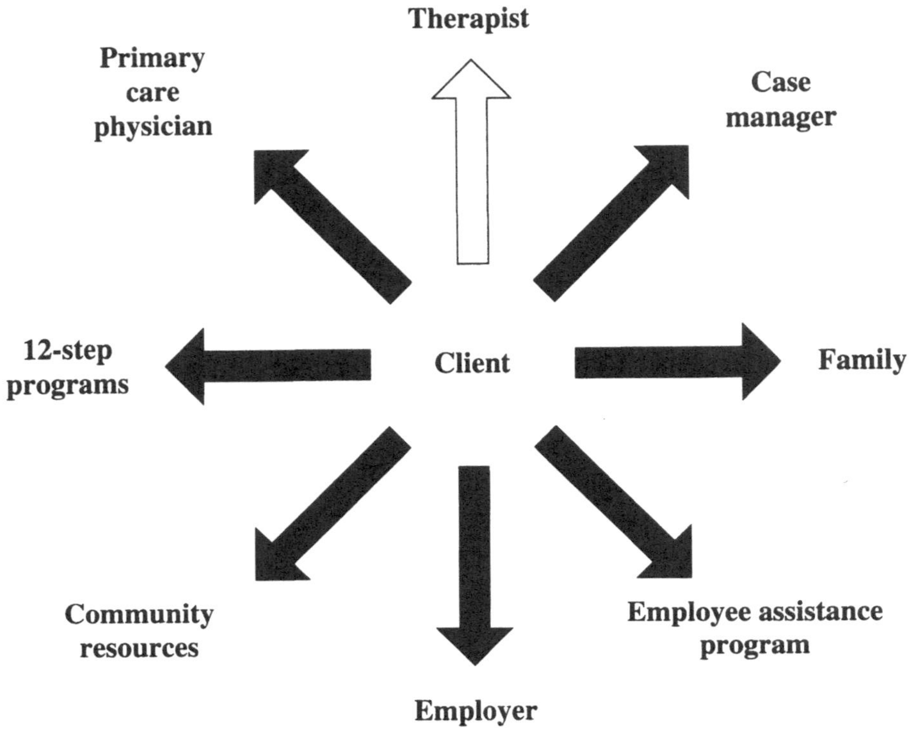

Q How are managed care panels going to be smaller when more providers are applying and the companies keep getting new contracts?

A Provider networks will change in size according to the companies' books of business. The companies may be adding providers in one geographic area, while reducing the network in another. But overall, it is estimated that national behavioral health networks will shrink by up to 20% during the next two to three years. Why will that happen? There are a number of contributing factors, including the managed care firm's decision to delete the provider based on profiling; the provider's dropping out of the system as the result of a decision to change his or her career or lifestyle, or because the number of referrals doesn't warrant remaining; or noncompliance with accreditation requirements or industry technological demands, such as quality management or electronic claims systems.

Q Sometimes there are clients who just can't be helped because they're not ready or don't acknowledge a need for treatment. What does a therapist do to keep this from reflecting badly on the managed care profile?

A When you as a therapist realize that the client match isn't good, there are three possible steps you might take: (1) Talk to the case manager for the managed care firm. Review the assessment and treatment plan and ask about options in your own treatment or about referring to another provider. (2) If the client isn't ready for therapy, determine whether there are self-help or community resources available in the interim. If there are, document the referral to the managed care firm. (3) If the client says he or she isn't open to therapy, make an appointment for a checkup three or six months later. Report that to the managed care firm as well.

Q What is provider profiling and how do the different companies determine who is a competent therapist?

EXHIBIT 2.4. What Managed Care Reviews.

Number of denials

Readmissions

Outcomes/patient satisfaction

Therapy approach

Case manager's experience

ALOS—average length of stay

Referral patterns—to more restrictive care, to less restrictive care, to community services

Number of incidents and reports

A Provider profiling is a system that allows the managed care firm to evaluate the provider's performance on a given number of cases over a period of time. (See Exhibit 2.4.) Does the provider consistently authorize treatment for 11 sessions regardless of diagnosis? Does the provider access community resources and self-help groups when appropriate? Is the provider cooperative when dealing with case managers? Most companies now factor in the level of acuity of patients being seen by particular providers, especially in light of Medicaid populations being added to most client mixes. Add to that clinical case review, quality assurance, and feedback from the beneficiary. The managed care company's goal is to identify providers who are good therapists and who are comfortable working within the confines of managed care, and to reward them with additional referrals.

The results of a recent pilot project released by the Merit Behavioral Care Corp. include these variables: case manager incident reports and red flags, suicides, unnecessary hospitalizations, efficient use of resources, a crisis-therapy approach with a targeted therapy focus, clinical outcomes, and patient satisfaction. U.S. Behavioral Health has a system whereby case managers do a dynamic rating of providers based on their more subjective opinions. The difficulty with this system is that the opinions of one case manager after a single bad interaction with a provider can skew the entire profile, even though performance may be high and patients may be satisfied.

Providers should routinely ask to review their profiles with case managers. Asking if your profile includes a new therapy group offering or extended office hours is a good way to involve a case manager in reviewing your profile—and it flags you as an active provider.

Q How is profiling different from credentialing?

A Profiling is a system that produces an image of the provider's performance within the managed care system over a period of time. Credentialing is the process of selecting and admitting providers to managed panels or systems. Profiling plays a key role in the recredentialing and selection of providers to remain on panels once in the system. See Exhibit 2.5 for selection, credentialing, and recredentialing criteria as described by John S. Montgomery, M.D., corporate medical director for Human Affairs International (Montgomery, 1995).

Q Can I look at my profile?

EXHIBIT 2.5. How Networks Are Built.

Provider Selection	Provider Recredentialing	Provider Credentialing
• Clinical philosophy • Quality of care • Managed care experience/attitude • Criteria for core selection • Collaborative relationship with network management	• Member satisfaction data • Quality indicator summaries • Complaint logs • Risk management issues • Provider outcomes • Provider profiling/ report cards • Clinical chart reviews	• Consistently administered criteria • Primary-source verification • Local credentialing committees • NCQA compliance

A The way the question is asked seems to have a lot to do with how it is answered. Demanding that a managed care firm release everything it knows about a provider doesn't usually win friends, or produce results. Instead, clinicians say they are most successful when they approach the case manager by asking to update their lists of specialties or to report changes in office locations or hours. The idea is to convey to the company that you want to make sure that your information is correct and up-to-date. This is a good time to ask to see your profile.

Updating is more important now than ever before. Managed care firms are purging inactive providers from their networks. Most are saying that it isn't worth the time and money to maintain files on providers who aren't receiving referrals. Credentialing costs at least $100, sometimes as much as $400, per provider, per year. Of course, providers don't receive referrals if they have inaccurate and dated profiles. Updating information with a new address, expanded hours, or added specialties can revive a sluggish profile and keep you in the system. Besides, it gives you a reason to talk with the case manager, and that's the best way to generate referrals.

Q I've heard that managed care companies rate providers on how quickly they can see patients. What is expected?

A The rule of thumb for most managed care firms is emergency telephone response within 30 minutes with clients seen the same day, appointment availability for urgent cases within 48 hours, and the ability to schedule routine appointments within five days. Standards proposed for managed behavioral health care firms by the National Committee on Quality Assurance (NCQA) focus on access and call for subscribers to be able to reach inpatient care within one hour and outpatient providers within 30 minutes; emergency visits must be scheduled within four hours of a referral call, urgent calls scheduled within 24 hours, and nonurgent visits within five business days. And managed care firms would be required to answer calls with a nonrecorded voice within 30 seconds. If implemented as expected, providers can expect those standards to be passed along to them by the companies.

Q I understand that some panels credential short-term providers and long-term providers. Please explain how this works, and the difference.

A There are a number of models used by the various companies. One firm credentials providers with strong diagnostic skills to do only assessments, referrals, and treatment for one to three sessions. Short-term providers for another firm see clients for up to eight sessions. Both call for quick assessment and referral to other resources—usually legal or financial counseling—if the problem doesn't really require behavioral health care.

If the client needs more treatment after the initial three or eight sessions, a referral is made to therapists who, because of their specialties or skills, will see the client for additional authorized sessions. Keep in mind that long-term therapy in these cases is usually no more than 15 or 20 sessions.

The idea is to discourage therapists from routinely entering treatment plans calling for long-term care. The managed care firm is able to use the assessing provider and the longer-term treating provider as a checks-and-balance system, using the assessment recommendations to monitor the treatment plan.

Merit Behavioral Care's Assessment, Referral and Counseling (ACR) group practices are good examples of this kind of system, where selected provider groups screen all patients for substance abuse problems. After evaluating the patient, the group practice either provides brief counseling or makes a referral within the network provider system.

Q Are there ever times when managed care will pay for long-term care?

A Yes. As managed care firms take on contracts for Medicaid and other public-sector clients, they are becoming acutely aware that some levels of severity cannot be treated with brief therapy. Managed care firms are most receptive to considering longer-term care for intractable or "brittle" disorders that require supportive work and medications (schizophrenia, bipolar). Psychiatrists who use treatment plans to show that a patient's condition is a direct result of a DSM-IV condition, and that the patient can be treated with psychotherapy at a lesser cost, are getting approval for requested sessions (Sabin, 1995). Managed care firms look closely at whether extended therapy can prevent hospitalizations.

Q Why are all these different panels demanding malpractice verification, state licensure verification, and national registry? It costs a lot of money. Why won't they accept copies of my documents?

A The managed care firms are liable for primary-source verification when they credential providers. Employer clients started to ask the managed care firms: How are you sure that what the provider is saying is true? And about 1% of providers have fudged on applications, with a handful of those cases widely reported, raising client anxiety.

Employers ask managed care firms:

- How do you know for certain that your providers have malpractice insurance?
- What if they just photocopy someone else's malpractice insurance, or white out their names and photocopy that?
- How are you sure that they haven't had major malpractice action taken against them?
- How are you sure that their state license hasn't been revoked since the time that you brought them on the panel?

All managed care firms accredited by the National Committee on Quality Assurance (NCQA) must conduct primary-source verification by outside companies at an average annual cost of $65 per provider for credentialing and up to $100 for recredentialing. HMOs have reported that compiling a credentialing folder of up to 30 pages takes an average of five hours at a cost of $300 to $400—a key reason for resistance to any-willing-provider mandates (Rovner,

1995). Several of the large carve-out firms, as members of the American Managed Behavioral Healthcare Association (AMBHA), may contract with a single vendor to do all first-level primary source verification (Gruttadaro, 1996). Providers would only have to provide documents once for credentialing by those member firms. Each member company would pay a fee for the service, and there is a good chance that providers would be charged also. Already, we're hearing of provider-sponsored behavioral health delivery systems charging $50 or $75 to offset the cost of primary source verification. (See Exhibit 2.6.)

Q What items would be included in the AMBHA credentialing?

A The credentialing would include the items required for the managed care firms to meet NCQA accreditation.* Among these are:

1. License and any state sanctions, restrictions, or limitations.
2. Work history.
3. Malpractice insurance and liability claims history.
4. National Practitioner Data Bank query.
5. Medicare/Medicaid sanctions.

Q What is the National Practitioner Data Bank?

A The National Practitioner Data Bank (NPDB) maintains information about malpractice insurance payments and policy status, state licensing board disciplinary actions, and malpractice awards involving all health care practitioners. It is primarily a flagging system for attaching derogatory actions to the files of licensed providers, including psychotherapists. Established under the Health Care Quality Improvement Act of 1986, the NPDB requires hospitals and other health care facilities to submit

***NCQA Guidelines and Standards for MCO Accreditation.* NCQA is a nonprofit organization that accredits and sets standards for managed care firms, primary-source-verification companies, and large provider group practices. Copies of guidelines and standards may be obtained by calling the NCQA at 202-955-3535.

EXHIBIT 2.6.
National Behavioral Healthcare Verification Services Flowchart.

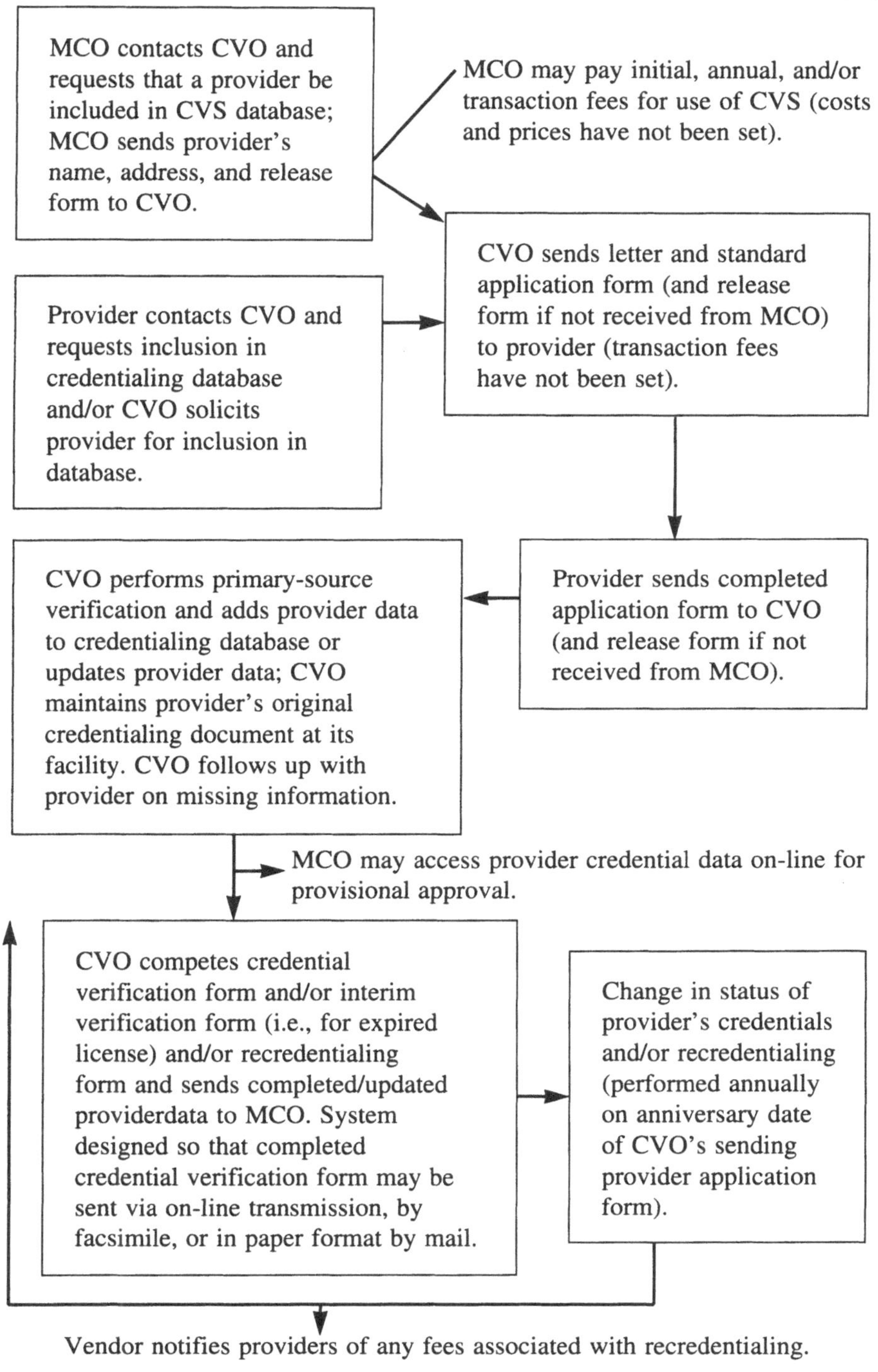

Source: Darcy Gruttadaro. Reprinted with permission.

reports within 15 days of an adverse action against a provider. State licensing boards, malpractice payers, and professional associations also are required to report disciplinary actions. Providers are issued NBPD identification numbers that allow them to check information in their file. The NCQA requires that managed care firms check NPDB files when credentialing providers. The NPDB Help Line number is 800-767-6732.

Q How can a practitioner manage managed care? There are so many kinds of review and forms to fill out that it becomes almost impossible to squeeze in business and clients. Is there a way to consolidate forms and procedures to make the provider's life easier?

A There's a very good chance that provider applications and credentialing will be streamlined soon. A trade group of companies specializing in managed mental health care—the AMBHA—is reviewing proposals to contract with a single vendor for standard credentialing of providers. It's unlikely that all companies would subscribe to the universal credentialing. But for those companies that do, providers would apply only once, using a single standard form. The companies would then select providers from the preapproved pool, individualizing networks to meet the specific needs of their employer clients. The advantage for participating companies would be lower administrative costs. There are a number of cooperative projects among managed care firms to share outcomes measurements and to set standards for care. It's more likely that accreditation standards being set by outside agencies—responding to employer demands—will define those standards. As firms are accredited, providers can expect those standards to filter down. For now, the most direct route to fewer forms and less oversight is capitation—an equally complex system and a riskier one.

CLINICAL DETAILS

Q What is care management?

A Care management refers to the clinical review of a client's diagnosis and treatment from the beginning to the end of an episode of care. This includes the authorization of benefit days within a specific time period. Care, or case, managers are expected to make recommendations and to act as a resource for the clinician in planning appropriate treatment within the constraints of the employee's benefit plan. Other case management responsibilities include triage, referral, evaluation of consumer needs and coordination of those needs with provider specialties, tracking of treatment progress, crisis intervention, and the handling of emergency calls.[†] The typical case manager in 15 of the largest managed behavioral health care firms is a registered nurse or a licensed master's-level clinician with three to 18 years of experience.[†]

Q How do I choose an outcomes measurement tool?

A Too many providers hesitate at measuring the results of their treatment because the concept seems expensive and involved. It doesn't have to be. Managed care firms, employers, and primary care referral sources are looking for easy-to-understand, comparative data that address patient functionality and satisfaction.

At least 50% of managed care firms responding to a 1995 survey by Mental Health Corporations of America, Inc., reported using outcomes measurements as a criterion for provider selection (*Contracting decisions,* 1995). Another 17% said they rely on the data to make referrals. *Practice Strategies* reported in its 1995 managed behavioral health care industry survey (Tuttle, 1995) that most larger carve-out firms measure outcomes internally, rarely shifting that responsibility to provider groups. Outcomes information from both groups and internal studies, however, was used by 70% of those firms when deciding which providers would remain on panels and the volume of referrals they would receive.

Best results are achieved when providers break out results by diagnosis and graph their findings to make them easy for payers to read. Tracking discharged patients at intervals of 3, 6, and 12 months indicates recidivism and continued functionality rates.

Some group practices buy standard tools and adapt them to include satisfaction questions asked at patient intake. The most important point is for providers to get started and to incorporate the results of their measurements in marketing materials. (See Appendix D for a listing of simple outcomes tools, with manufacturers' addresses and telephone numbers.)

[†] *Case manager qualifications in AMBHA member companies,* AMBHA, 700 13th Street, NW, Suite 950, Washington, DC 20005; phone 202-434-4565. Survey reports are available for $10.

Q Please give details, length, and content of what should be in a treatment plan.

A Treatment plan specifications vary with managed care firms. One thing no managed care firm wants is an exhaustive psychosocial history. The ideal treatment plan includes identifying information—age, sex, marital status—and then a short narrative that discusses the presenting problem. For example: "This is a 38-year-old, self-referred Asian male. He is experiencing an extreme amount of depression. His symptoms include insomnia, midnight awakening, decreased libido, and/or decreased energy and ability to enjoy life." (See Exhibit 2.7.)

Then outline the proposed plan for treating those symptoms. It should include details of who will be coming for sessions, what his or her problem is, what you want to do about the problem, how you plan to do it, and how long you think it will take. For example: "Mr. Jones, a 42-year-old African-American male, referred himself with symptoms of severe depression. I will refer him for medication consultation, look at specific precipitants and continued symptoms of the depression, and try to help resolve the depression through cognitive behavioral therapy. I believe this will take 10 to 12 sessions."

Most providers who have problems with treatment plans are reluctant to share information about the client. The company is looking for information that verifies clinical necessity under the employer's benefit plan. Then the provider requests the number of sessions that seems appropriate. The content of the treatment, legibly written on the company's preferred form, is more important than length. Read companies' provider manuals for samples, or ask the case manager for a sample of that firm's ideal treatment plan. (See Exhibit 2.8.)

Q Why should therapy time be used to involve the patient in writing a treatment plan just to satisfy managed care companies?

A There's a good deal of provider debate over this question. Providers coming from community mental health centers and public sector backgrounds are accustomed to writing treatment plans and are comfortable with the process. Advocates of treatment plans say they're not just paper trails, but a tool to make patients active participants in their treatment. Some

EXHIBIT 2.7. Ten Steps to Treatment Planning.

Producing a written treatment plan is a necessity for most clinicians working in private practice. The more readily that it can be integrated into the practice routine, the less time it will take. Time is a precious commodity for the busy clinician. Careful and comprehensive treatment planning will lead to a smoother ride on the managed care road.

1. **Comprehensive overview:** Give a full profile of the patient, including reasons and necessity for treatment. Include history, symptoms, diagnosis, and focus of treatment.

2. **Goals and progress:** State treatment goals in measurable terms. Set target times for goals. Link improvement to specific interventions and detail levels of progress leading to discharge.

3. **Action:** Reflect the thinking, planning, and action steps taken by the therapist with the patient. Think brief therapy in terms of promoting change.

4. **Timeliness:** Coordinate treatment planning with requests for authorization and billing for services. Late treatment plans are often the cause of frustrating telephone calls and repeated requests for paperwork.

5. **Benefit awareness:** Know the limits and specifics of the patient's benefits plan before submitting a treatment plan. If the benefits only cover three to five sessions, requesting authorization for 25 sessions is unrealistic.

6. **Adjunctive services and support:** Consider other levels of care and incorporate those into the treatment plan. These should include hospitalization, day treatment, intensive outpatient treatment, medication, group therapy, 12-step programs, parenting classes, and other community self-help resources.

7. **Liaison with other professionals:** Indicate involvement of other professionals in the treatment process where appropriate.

8. **Crisis and potential red flags:** Show understanding of potential crisis situations and the need for crisis intervention and a willingness to involve the case manager in those decisions.

9. **Chemical dependency treatment:** Address the need for evaluation and intervention for chemical dependency issues, with appropriate referrals to inpatient, intensive outpatient, or 12-step programs.

10. **Copies:** Always keep copies of treatment plans and authorizations. Save yourself headaches from lost paperwork and treatment plans that never reach case managers.

Source: Scott Harris. *Treatment Planning: A managed care guide to the rules of the road.* Reprinted with permission.

EXHIBIT 2.8. Example of a Completed Treatment Planning Form.

Narrative: This is a 38-year old Asian male who is self-referred. He reports being very depressed. Symptoms include insomnia, midnight awakening, and decreased libido.

Patient Name: William Lee **Social Security #:** 555-55-5555
Date: 4/30/97 **Provider's Name:** M.C. Provider, LCSW, BCD
Telephone Number: (555) 555-5555
Primary Care Physician's Name: Dr. John Gatekeeper
Date of Initial Session: 5/31/96 **Subscriber(s) in Treatment:**

Employee: **x**	Sex: **M**	Age: **38**
Spouse:	Sex:	Age:
Child:	Sex:	Age:

Statement of Subscriber's Problem(s). (Be specific. Describe in terms of functional impairment and/or personal discomfort. Indicate areas of life affected.)

1. Patient is recently separated from wife of 18 years and four children
2. Insomnia
3. Inability to focus on work for more that 45 minutes at a time
4. Prescribed Prozac by his primary care physician
5. Feels extremely hopeless; denies suicidality

Relevant Psychosocial and Work History: (Include levels of adaptive functioning.)

Mr. Lee is an architect who has felt successful at all that he's attempted in his life. He views divorce as an extreme failure and did not want a separation. He has been intensely involved in church activities with his family and feels that he cannot now attend church. His parents reside in the area and judge him quite harshly for his inability to manage his family. He has never lived alone. He left his parents' home to marry and live with his wife. He has worked at his firm for 15 years and is up for a partnership.

Alcohol or Drug Abuse Problem? Yes _x_ No ___ If yes, describe:

Although he has been a social drinker, since his divorce Mr. Lee has consumed a bottle of wine each evening for the past month. He feels perpetually hung over. This may bear on his inability to focus at work. His father has a history of alcoholism and binge drinking.

Page 1

Subscriber has primary care physician? Yes _x_ No ___

Contacted? Yes _x_ No ___

This was a referral from the primary care physician. I asked client to sign a release of information form, which he did. I contacted the physician to confirm his attendance and to consult re: medication type and dosage that he is currently taking.

Medical History, Concurrent Medical Problems and Treatment: (Indicate any communication with physicians involved, include dates.)

Client is severely hypertensive. Medication is Prinivil, dosage is 30 mg x 1 daily. Physician states that there are no adverse interactions between Prinivil and Prozac. Concerns are the interactions of alcohol with Prinivil and Prozac.

Psychotropic Medication: (Indicate physician, medication, follow-up, include dates.)

Prozac 5 mg b.i.d., prescribed by primary care physician—physician requires quarterly visit for follow-up. Last follow-up on 4/12/97.

Planned Therapeutic Interventions:

1. Primary approach: crisis intervention, supportive intervention.

   Focused symptom reduction or behavioral change x assessment and referral only.
2. Referral to chemical dependency two-week education and insight program for assessment.
3. Psychotherapy to address issues of abandonment and low self-esteem (10 sessions) following C.D. treatment.
4. Address issues of perceived failure.
5. Refer to pastor for counseling, re: returning to church.
6. One session with spouse to assess potential for marital therapy.
7. Reassessment of therapeutic dosage of Prozac or other medication with group psychiatrist.

Diagnosis:
DSM-IV:

Axis I: Major depression
Axis II: None
Axis III: None
Axis IV: (Psychosocial Stressors) Severe
Axis V: **Current GAF:** 75

providers, burdened by paperwork and squeezed by low rates and mounting referrals, have shaved five minutes from sessions just for this purpose. So, the session is described as 45 minutes of therapy.

Therapists who are comfortable working with managed care firms defend treatment plans, saying patients like the involvement in their treatment and that the plans lead to more focused care. "Most private practitioners 10 years ago did not even think about a treatment plan—they might or might not have had one in their head," says Evelyn M. Frye, a Nashville, Tenn., psychologist who owns a multidisciplinary group practice (Defino, 1996). "Long term, it should have a positive impact on the practice of psychotherapy and mental health."

Q What is utilization review?

A The therapist provides the case manager with information necessary to support the authorization for continued treatment. The initial review is the one done after you've seen the client for the first time. You call in and discuss the problem and propose a plan for treatment. It involves sharing of confidential information. Providers should make sure that clients sign an information release form as part of their intake procedure, even if they signed a global release when accepting coverage under the managed care plan.

Q What is authorization?

A Authorization of treatment by the managed care organization confirms the client's and therapist's rights to claim reimbursement from the company for a limited number of sessions during a coverage period. One caveat: Authorization does not guarantee that therapists will be paid. If the client is not eligible for coverage, the payment won't be made, or the provider might have to refund the money under retroactive deletion clauses. Be aware, authorization does not guarantee that you will be paid. If the client is not eligible—for example, if he or she is no longer working or has stopped making dependent premium payments—the authorization is void.

This shifts the burden to the provider to be able to verify benefit coverage before treating the patient. We regularly hear of providers willing to spend 20 to 30 minutes on intake, placing calls to insurers and employers to verify coverage before the first visit. Benefit verification should become easier as providers go on-line with software that connects them to managed care firms and insurers for automatic verification. When contracting with managed care firms, providers should ask how coverage is verified: How much time elapses between a plan action, such as removing an employee from the plan, and when that information is entered into the insurance system? The lag is usually at least 30 days, and treatment authorized during that time won't be covered. Notify the client that he or she is financially responsible for noncovered services.

Q Why are additional authorizations needed for continued treatment?

A Treatment outside of the plan agreed to by the clinician and case manager requires authorization or the company won't pay. Not only that, but under some contracts, treatment outside the benefit plan can jeopardize the employee's total benefit coverage. There are emergency situations that can call for unauthorized care, or new situations can arise during therapy that call for changing the treatment plan. The key is to stay in close communication with the case manager. Don't treat and then ask, unless it is an absolute emergency. And in those cases, try to reach the case manager as quickly as possible and document efforts in the clinical records.

Exhibit 2.9 takes a humorous look at authorization.

Q Why do clients think they have, say, 50 allowed sessions, whereas the provider is only authorized to provide a lesser number?

A Managing the amount of care that is appropriate to the diagnosis with the patient's actual needs is the cornerstone of managed behavioral health care. The plan may provide coverage for a maximum number of sessions, but carte blanche entitlement to each and every session is what triggered employers to begin trimming benefit packages and managing care.

It is the managed care firm's job to "manage" the utilization of benefits and to authorize payment based on clinical necessity. Clients don't always understand their benefits package. Again, this shifts the burden to the provider to discuss the benefits package with the patient, and to explain that the maximum will not be authorized automatically, and that the diagnosis, treatment plan, and discussion with the case manager will determine the level of eligibility.

EXHIBIT 2.9.

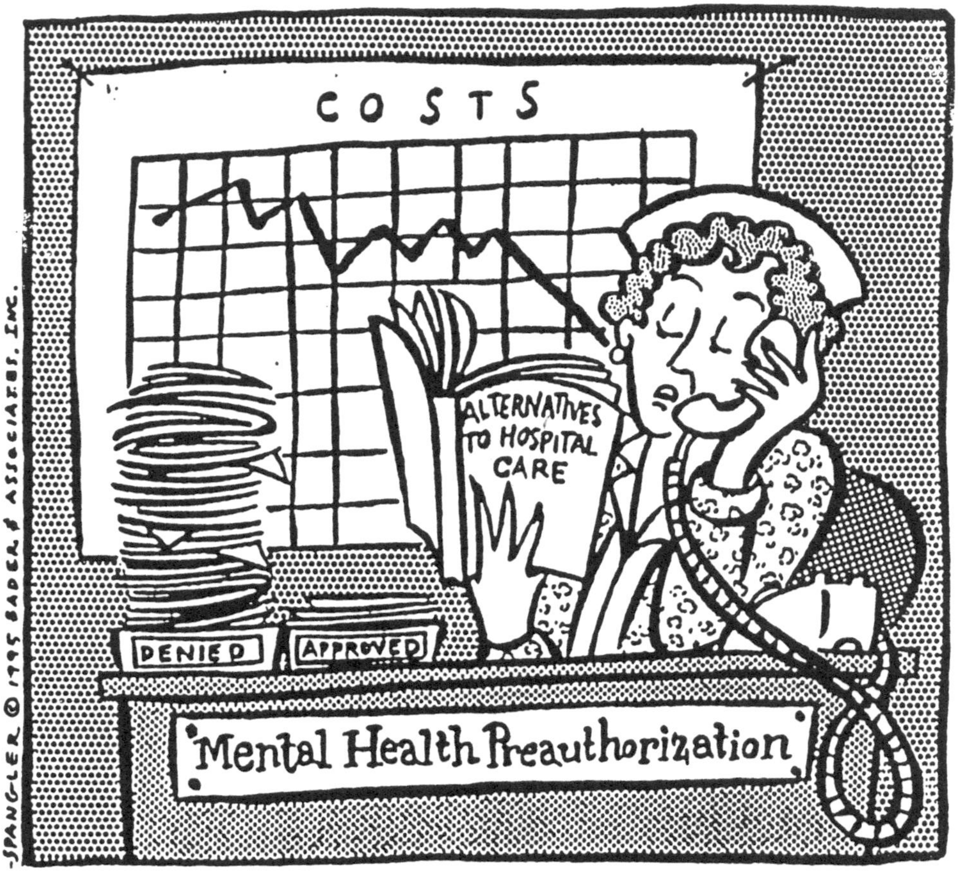

"How can you be sure you're depressed, Sir? Why not go out for dinner and a movie and see if you feel better?"

Source: Health System Leader. Courtesy of Capitol Publications, Alexandria, VA.

Q **Doesn't work with the brief model espoused by managed care force you to abandon your clients?**

A Patient abandonment is failure to ensure appropriate care, or to make the appropriate referral when you terminate with a patient. It is important to document issues and concerns about a client to ensure that he or she receives the appropriate level of benefit. If you believe that a patient needs additional services and is at risk if not seen, you have at least three options:

1. Appeal the decision to terminate benefits and continue to see the client until you have completed the appeal.
2. Transfer the patient to a private-pay status at the rate that the managed care company paid you or at your sliding-scale rate.
3. Transfer the client to the appropriate community resource, private agency, or group practice. Create a form that documents your referral (such as an emergency referral form) and get your client to sign that he or she understands the referral. Follow up to ensure that the referral has been accomplished.

Q What happens if the case manager doesn't agree? Is there a way to advocate for a client without being dropped from a panel?

A There definitely is a way to advocate for a client. Most managed care companies have appeal procedures. Ask to review those procedures before signing a provider contract. Use these procedures judiciously—not because you think that a client who has a 20-session benefit should get 40 sessions. That's not possible. Instead, rely on appeals when you think the case manager who is handling the case is not listening carefully and isn't understanding, or when you need to clarify a treatment misunderstanding. Ethically, it is your obligation as the person providing sessions to advocate for the client and to go up the appeals ladder.

And it is your responsibility as a network provider to do that in a way that doesn't undermine case managers. One approach would be: "I understand what you're saying, but I need to advocate for my client, so I really need to take this to the next level. I think it's important to appeal this. Can you help direct me through the appropriate channels?" Appealing becomes an important legal issue if you think that essential care is being denied. In a number of lawsuits, including *Wickline v. The State of California*, courts have held that clinicians who fail to appeal when appropriate are liable for malpractice.

Providers who use the appeals process wisely don't need to worry about panel security. Railing at the case manager and the person's supervisor is not part of the procedure. When filing a legitimate appeal, document each step in writing. Again, most managed care firms—the ones with which you will want to do business—will have an appeals committee that includes your peers to review any suspected retaliation. Most contracts allow for binding arbitration as a last resort.

Outside of the managed care firm's system, providers can appeal to their state insurance commission's managed care division.

Q What do case managers do when they receive planning forms?

A Upon receiving the forms, they confirm the diagnosis, look at changes or revisions to the treatment plan, look at the status of the client, document progress or the reason why the client is not progressing, and review the termination goals and plan. Payment is authorized if the paperwork agrees with the plan.

Q In chemical dependency treatment, when group therapy and inpatient intensive bombardment are needed to break denial (7 to 10 days of inpatient care), why is this not respected?

A When managed care companies were developing, they asked about the need for 28-day programs and were told that that amount of inpatient time was needed to allow patients to be confronted and educated.

Next, the companies asked whether the intensive inpatient work could be shifted to residential treatment, so that patients still would be out of their homes but in a less expensive setting than an acute-care hospital. Studies reported the same outcomes in residential care.

The next step was to put all of the psychoeducational pieces on an outpatient or day treatment basis with a longer episode of care. Effectiveness in those settings is still being reviewed. The bottom line is that managed care firms have the task of finding the least-restrictive, most cost-effective way of delivering all levels of care.

PROVIDER RELATIONS

Q How can a case manager help providers?

A Not all case managers will be helpful, just as not all providers are polite or receptive to suggestions about therapy approaches. But a good relationship with a case manager can be the therapist's best resource. The case manager knows the benefit plan inside and out, and has access to the client's history—both useful pieces of information in producing a successful treatment plan. Case managers are good troubleshooters, and good advocates for flexing benefits to meet a treatment plan calling for alternative levels of care, and they will provide you with new referrals.

Q What about case managers who are clerks or secretaries with no clinical training? How can they handle a patient they've never seen when they don't even know the terminology of therapy?

A It's a fact that a number of early managed care firms used nonclinicians for telephone utilization review. The reality today, however, is that most major managed care companies are staffed by psychologists, social workers, marriage and family therapists, and psychiatrists who do peer review and make decisions based on clinical information provided by the treating therapist.

In some managed care firms, the only person with whom a therapist ever has contact is a clerk, even though a clinician has reviewed the treatment plan. The problem is due, in part, to the rapid growth of such managed care firms, with case managers, secretaries, and clerks screening thousands of plans for medical necessity. That's troubling for therapists who aren't comfortable discussing cases with clerks and secretaries. Some companies are using computer-scanned bubble charts for noting symptoms and authorizing early sessions so that the provider skips the clerical encounter until the case reaches a clinician review. You have the right to speak to a clinician.

Case manager duties vary among large managed care firms, as reported by AMBHA in a membership survey. The roles and responsibilities of case managers as described by 15 large companies were the review of authorizations; coordination of and liaison with primary care providers and network providers; triage, referral, and evaluation; monitoring for member follow-through, coordination of care, and discharge planning; crisis assessment and emergency calls; catastrophic case management; initial assessment; and arranging transportation and alternative care.

The typical case manager in the AMBHA member companies is a registered nurse or licensed master's-level clinician with 3 to 14 years of experience. In 13 of the 15 companies responding, all denials of service are made by a medical doctor. In 12 of the 15 companies, case managers are supervised or trained by a doctor. Three of the firms require master's-level clinical training for intake workers, while eight accept bachelor's level workers with customer service experience (*Case Manager Qualifications,* 1996).

Q Will managed care pay for treating other problems when a client has a chemical dependency problem?

A A number of large employers, including IBM, discovered that they were spending a lot of money to treat anxiety, depression, and marital problems—and then were spending more money to treat contributing alcohol and chemical dependencies. Managed care firms, responding to those employer needs, now generally expect providers to screen for and treat addictions before they will approve treatment plans for other diagnoses. Most have criteria for chemical dependency screenings. Check your provider manual and talk with the case manager.

Q What is triangulation? Why do I get into trouble when I advocate for my client?

A Triangulation refers to providers stepping outside the authorized appeals process to encourage the patient to protest the managed care firm's handling of care. Remember that the managed care firm's job is to authorize and manage care within the benefit plan as approved by the employer. There is an appeals process for both the provider and the employee when they disagree with either the level of coverage or the managed care firm's interpretation of the benefit plan. Providers typically do not have problems when they follow the appeals procedure. Many problems occur when the provider fails to read the contract for services, the provider manual, and the company's treatment guidelines. That means the provider is also likely to begin the appeals process without first becoming familiar with the required steps.

In most cases, the patient isn't fully aware of why the case manager has denied additional sessions and the provider may be disregarding the benefit plan and purposely not explaining the benefit limits to the patient. The better course of action is to make the patient aware of what his or her benefits will cover, discuss the treatment plan with the patient, review the appeals process, and then help the patient explore options to help pay for additional treatment, if it is in fact warranted.

Q What are some of the things that providers do that can really screw up the relationship with a managed care company?

A There are several things that can really get providers into trouble with managed care firms. Here is the list of top picks by one the authors (Dianne Rush Woods):

1. **Being rude to intake coordinators and case managers.** Case managers take rude comments personally and tend to avoid providers who blame them for changes under managed care. The golden rule applies here: Do unto others as you would have them do unto you. Using the telephone line as a buffer, providers often vent their frustrations on case managers and utilization reviewers. Often, those reviewers are clinical peers, licensed as psychologists, social workers, marriage and family therapists, or psychiatrists. Managing the verbal relationship with managed care employees should be a priority for providers.

   It may seem that you're making rude comments to a faceless stranger, but utilization reviewers do get promoted and they drink coffee with people who can affect your panel status. Woods shares this example: "I was the director of provider relations at a large managed care company when I interviewed a provider applicant whom I thought was quite personable. Later, I learned that the candidate had been very rude and obnoxious to my staff. None of this came through to me, but because my staff had reported it, I chose not to credential the provider. So it's really important to know that the way you act toward one individual in an organization can travel to people who have the power to turn off the juice."

2. **Being tardy with reports.** Providers who are consistently late in submitting documentation have problems with managed care. Submitting documentation for sessions that have already been completed can stop payments.

3. **Being unwilling to go the extra mile.** Case managers find it easy to forget about the providers who are never available for crises, or who can never help out by taking a late Friday or early Saturday session.

   However, providers who are available are easily remembered for referrals. Just mentioning the name of one of those providers drew this response from a provider relations director. "Oh yes, Betty. She is always available. She is always responsive. She is one of our top people because she shows that she cares about us and about our clients."

4. **Submitting illegible treatment plans.** If case managers can't read the treatment plan, they can't authorize sessions or payment. Providers who are just naturally sloppy writers should consider taking advantage of electronic technology that allows treatment plans to be transmitted over a modem directly into the managed care system, or as a fax.

5. **Hospitalizing patients without consulting with the managed care firm.** Providers who consistently hospitalize or go to a higher level of care rather than consulting with the managed care company to agree on an appropriate level of care are seen as being difficult.

6. **Putting the patient in the middle of disagreements.** Providers who go around the case manager, or who use the patient to manipulate the system, are not popular. "Your inadequate policy with this company keeps me from providing your care," is an example of a statement to a patient that would place a provider at odds with the company. That type of remark sets up an adversarial relationship *through* the client. Providers who advocate for themselves and their clients are respected, and should be respected. An example of a better way to communicate with the patient is, "I think you're going to need additional sessions and we're going to have to look at your benefits closely to see if we can get payment approval for those. I'll suggest a treatment plan to your managed care company, and once that has been reviewed, we'll discuss the options available."

CONTINUUM OF CARE

Q What is a continuum of care?

A It's the entire range of care, from community self-help groups to inpatient care spread across a delivery system that optimally affords payers and patients one-stop shopping; it is also referred to as vertical integration. A continuum of services must be provided by an integrated delivery system through a staff or network model (Donahue & Wirecki, 1995). The delivery system could be driven by a facility, hospital, or group practice. The current thinking is that patients enter the system at the least restrictive level of care and are stepped up to more intensive care, if needed.

Initially, the interim-level programs were developed as "step downs" from inpatient care to less expensive, less restrictive alternatives. Capitated contracting is essential to managing care across the continuum. Common goals throughout a continuum of care are to base treatment decisions on DSM-IV diagnoses; to maintain a level of functionality with the aim of keeping the employee or student on the job or in school, or returning the patient to either as soon as possible; and to ease the movement of patients from one level to the next. Components of a full continuum might include prevention, self-help, community resources and support groups, 12-step programs, 24-

hour crisis lines, mobile crisis intervention, in-home counseling teams, crisis groups, outpatient psychotherapy/medication, therapy groups, intensive outpatient (IOP) care, partial hospitalization, inpatient crisis stabilization, 23-hour beds, inpatient care, and aftercare (*The Continuum,* 1995). (See Exhibit 2.10.)

Q What defines partial hospitalization?

A A partial hospitalization program offers treatment at the same level as inpatient care, but without the overnight stay. It is often a step down from crisis intervention, 23-hour beds, or inpatient care. Most programs are structured for 6 to 8 hours daily, 5 to 7 days per week. As with intensive outpatient programs, treatment focuses on group therapy and includes family involvement, but also includes a clinical evaluation, psychopharmacology, and discharge planning. Patients can be stepped down to IOP programs. (The AABHC sets standards and guidelines for partial programs, and was instrumental in winning CHAMPUS approval for partial programs run by group practices. For information, contact Mark Knight, Executive Director, Association for Ambulatory Behavioral Healthcare, Outcomes Project, 901 N. Washington Street, Ste. 600, Alexandria, VA 23314; phone 703-836-2274.)

Q What is intensive outpatient treatment?

A Intensive outpatient treatment is less intensive than partial hospitalization, but more intensive than standard outpatient care. As part of the continuum of care, it is a step down from inpatient, partial hospitalization, crisis intervention, or 23-hour bed treatment. Most programs average two to three hours daily, for three to five days per week. Structured programs vary for adolescent, adult psychiatric, adult chemical dependency, and geriatric patients. Most include case management and group therapy combinations of occupational, vocational, and recreational therapies; 12-step programs; and individual treatment. Fees for IOPs can be as low as $150 per day, compared with inpatient costs of $500 to $800 a day. The IOP program at American Day Treatment Centers of Annapolis, MD, for example, includes mandatory Saturday morning sessions involving family members and three other days of treatment that include expressive, psychoeducational, and group therapy. Patients are admitted based on DSM-IV diagnosis and ability to function in a work or school setting while still needing treatment through a structured program.

EXHIBIT 2.10. Continuum of Care.

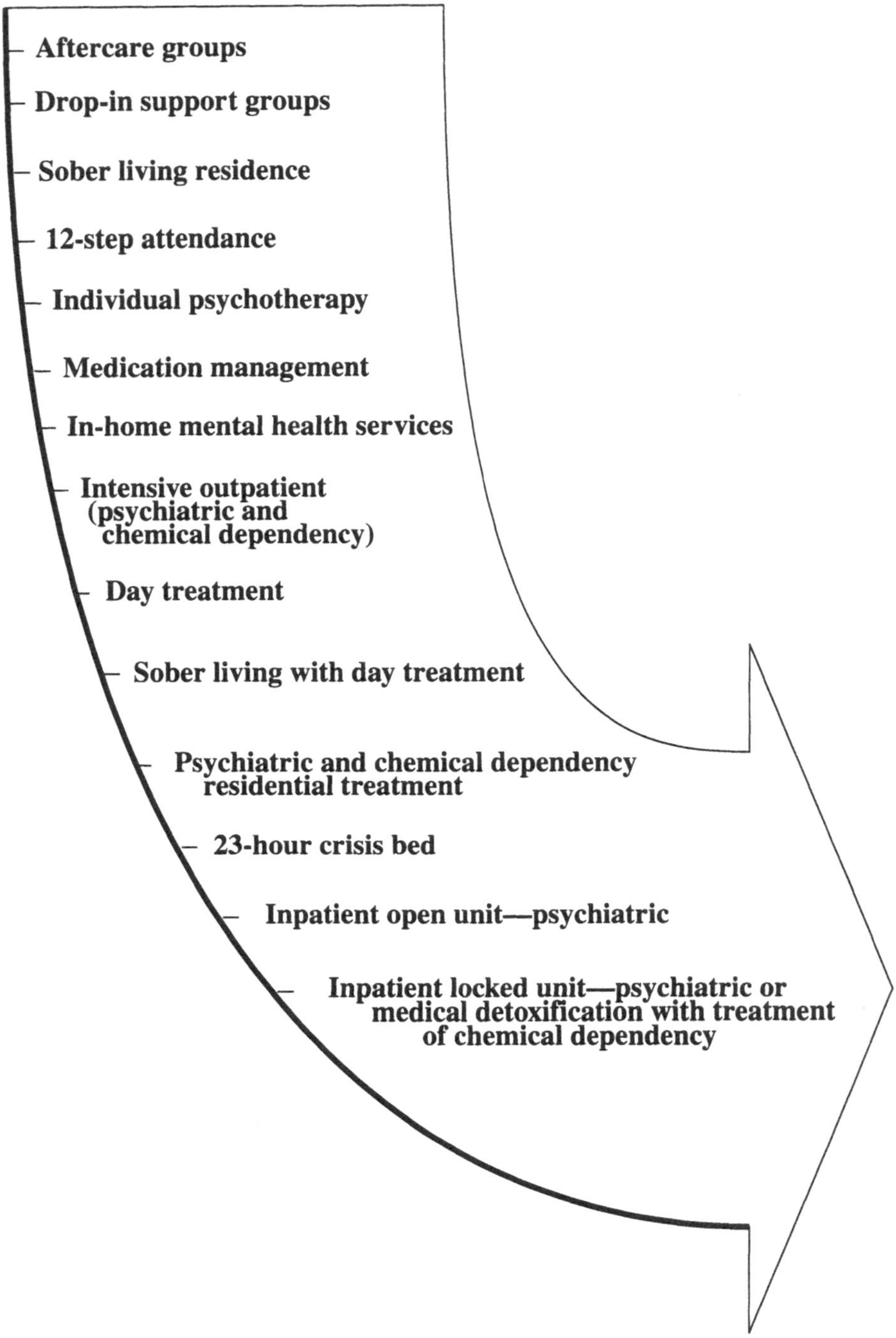

Q What is disease management? Where can one find guidelines that outline what to expect with disease management?

A Disease management means focusing on specific diagnoses and diseases and looking at them on the continuum that includes medical and behavioral health care components. The American Psychiatric Association has guidelines and the American Psychological Association provides information on how to review and handle plans that support the disease state management approach. Disease management templates have been developed for cardiac rehabilitation, diabetes, cancer, and the human immunodeficiency virus (HIV). Additional templates have been developed, or are in various stages of development, for anxiety and depression. In most cases, these include psychopharmaceutical products and talk therapy several steps into a treatment process initiated by the primary care physician. Among companies developing depression guidelines are Value Health Science, Greenstone Healthcare Solutions, Eli Lilly and Company, and Johnson & Johnson.

CONTRACT ISSUES

Q What is the most frequent cause for a provider being dropped from a panel?

A There are common reasons for terminating a provider, although managed care firms seldom cite them because most contracts contain no-cause termination clauses. That means that the company can drop the provider without giving a reason for doing so. A number of states have passed "right-to-know" legislation that will require managed care firms to tell providers in writing why they are rejected or dropped from a panel.

While unstated, the most common reason for releasing a provider from a network contract involves dual relationships. This includes inappropriate business, sexual, and other personal/professional relationships with current or former clients. It is usually revealed through routine recredentialing or the initial credentialing of a provider. If allegations were made in the past that have been proved false, it is important to report this on the application because such allegations are screened for thoroughly.

The second most common reason is disparagement of the managed care firm by the contracted provider. This includes providers who blame the managed care company for treatment of a patient as outlined in the employer's benefit package.

Managed care firms also drop providers who are rude to their case managers, or who call employers to complain about the company rather than using the company's appeals process.

Another reason might be perpetrating insurance fraud, such as signing documents indicating that services have been provided when they in fact have not, or that treatment was provided by someone other than the actual treating therapist. Charging the companies for missed appointments and refusing to collect patient copayments can also lead to dismissals.

Q What do I do if I am dropped from a panel?

A If the notice from the panel does not indicate a reason, contact the company's provider relations department to find out why you were removed from its network listing. Then check your contract to see if the company followed its provider agreements on terms for dropping providers and for notifying providers of its actions. Most early managed care contracts do allow for no-cause removal of network providers. A number of states, however, have passed any-willing-provider legislation or managed care regulations that include guidelines for how clinicians are selected, dropped from referral lists, and notified of the companies' actions. Ask your state insurance commissioner for copies of state regulations and compare them with your agreements.

The key issue that clinicians face when dropped from panels is the possible abandonment of current patients. Most managed care firms will allow providers to continue to see clients already in treatment, and, in many cases, the provider will be paid for those additional sessions at his or her usual and customary fee rather than at the negotiated reduced fee. Appeal the decision and request a written explanation for why you were dropped from the panel.

Q What should providers consider before signing with a specific managed care company?

A They should ask themselves: Am I willing to accept as payment what the company is willing to pay, including the co-payment? Am I willing to complete and submit the forms? Am I willing to comply with requirements for accessing the benefit, even if it is administered by the MCO? Am I willing to include a third party in the review process? Am I willing to submit my assessment and goals for treatment to a case manager? Am I willing to accept recommendations from that third party?

Ask to see a copy of the proposed contract and review it carefully. Also, ask for a copy of the company's provider manual, appeals process, and treatment guidelines. Make sure that you can live with the company's policies before you sign up. (See Exhibit 2.11.)

Q Do I need written permission from the patient in order to release clinical information to the managed care firm?

EXHIBIT 2.11. Tips for Reviewing Managed Care Firms.

- Ask the company for a copy of its contract to review. Request a copy of the contract manual, including the appeals process and guidelines for submitting claims and other required forms.
- Ask for a client list. Some companies routinely issue them with contracts. Others put together panels of providers for use in marketing to employer contracts.
- Ask for a ZIP code breakdown on the company's covered lives, and the pattern of referrals to providers during the last year.
- What are the assignment rights? Could the network be "sold" or "rented" to another company without your knowledge?
- What is the termination agreement? How can you get out, and can the company drop you without cause?
- What does the hold-harmless clause involve? Does your malpractice carrier cover any liability shifted to you under the contract?
- Can you self-refer, or refer out of the network?
- Is the discount structure based on volume?
- What kind of reports are required? Can your office staff handle them?
- Ask the managed care company for references of network providers. Call them and talk about their experience with the company.
- Ask that all of your clients be "bundled" to one case manager.
- Ask for the business. Ask for one or two patients on a trial basis. Then show your results.

A Yes, the information release form is one of the intake forms that the client signs at the first session. If clients do not want clinical information released to the third-party payer, providers should be prepared to review benefit requirements with the client and to offer possible alternatives, including private payment, or an outside referral if accepting private payment would jeopardize the managed care contract. While managed care firms generally provide release forms for their enrollees, all providers should make sure that a standard release form is part of their intake package.

Q **Is it best not to document services provided in order to ensure the patient's confidentiality?**

A Poor documentation of the treatment, patient complaints, supervision, or the patient's financial agreement can result in legal difficulties for the provider. If the patient complains, you need to be able to refer to your notes for your own information. Managed care contracts specify that providers are expected to keep appropriate client files for a specified period. As managed care firms comply with national accrediting standards, providers can expect periodical on-site audits of client files.

Q **How can a managed care firm audit my records?**

A Most information release forms and provider contracts from managed care firms include a statement to the effect that the company has the right to inspect clinical records periodically in order to ensure compliance with confidentiality and record-keeping requirements. While only one in 5,000 contracted providers has experienced record audits in the past, that situation is changing rapidly in response to accreditation requirements. Some companies will inspect records of up to 10% of their network providers, while the rule of thumb for others will be to audit records of high-volume providers—those receiving at least 5% of referrals in a given geographic area (Tuttle, 1996). Most inspect according to standard NCQA requirements for legible handwriting, identification of patient and date of treatment on each page, patient history, progress notes, screening for substance abuse or high-risk potential for it, signed release forms by patients, reports to primary care provider, and next scheduled appointment.

Q What about confidentiality? Isn't it automatically breached when I speak with a case manager? And don't case managers often pass the information on to employers?

A This is the most frequently asked ethical and legal question. Remembering that there are laws that bind what an individual, group, or mental health company can do in terms of confidential communication helps. Managed health care companies must abide by the same rigorous state and federal confidentiality laws that govern the individual provider. The managed care company acts as the insurance company. The company provides information release forms that, when signed by the client, allow the company to receive information that is used to validate the need for treatment. In order to receive payment, you are obligated to share a treatment plan and progress notes with the managed care firm.

The case managers at the managed care companies are required to sign complex statements ensuring their adherence to confidentiality. The companies have complicated computerized security systems to ensure confidentiality. Can it be violated? Certainly that can happen. As mentioned earlier, the only absolute guarantee of confidentiality is private pay under an assumed name.

Q What about fax/data transfers? This seems the ultimate breach of confidentiality.

A The choice to send information by facsimile transmission is truly up to the clinician. It is clearly the faster way to get data to the managed care firm. But providers should be clear about the managed care firm's policy for receiving faxes. Is the line dedicated? Is the fax machine located in a locked room with limited personnel access? Who receives the faxes and delivers them to the case manager? Has that person signed a confidentiality agreement? If the standards do not meet your standards, then do not fax documents. Be prepared to use second-day mail and overnight delivery services for rapid response.

Use a cover-sheet that indicates that the information is confidential, and that anyone receiving it by mistake should notify you and destroy the document. Use only the patient's Social Security number or an assigned number in faxed communications. And in your patient intake materials include a release form allowing you to use facsimile transmittals.

Q What happens if I conduct several groups and allow managed care patients to pay out of pocket? By doing so, I can save their maximum allowed sessions for individual care that can be spaced out, or for continuing group therapy after individual sessions have been used.

A Read your provider contract carefully, and suggest that the client also read his or her coverage manual carefully. Look for "outside-of-benefit" clauses that say that as a contract provider you may not see patients for sessions not covered under benefits. Providing services outside of the benefit plan defeats the company's motive of controlling costs by managing utilization. Remember, the managed care firm is going to want a treatment history as part of the treatment plan. Some managed care firms are willing to flex benefits to allow providers to substitute two sessions of group therapy for a single individual session, or to transfer inpatient dollars to cover less expensive outpatient services. That has to do with the employer benefits plan. It really is wise to talk with the managed care firm before working outside of the contract.

Q What about hold-harmless clauses?

A "Get rid of them," suggests Barton Bernstein, a Texas attorney who works with mental health providers (Bernstein, 1993). His contention is that hold-harmless clauses make providers the insurers of managed care. When providers sign contracts containing hold-harmless clauses, they are essentially agreeing to release the managed care firm from responsibility for treatment decisions. Many malpractice carriers won't cover providers who sign them. "You don't have to do anything wrong to run up a hefty bill," says Bernstein. "Just get sued and have to defend it."

At the very least, insist on dual indemnification. In other words, the company releases you from liability for its actions as well.

REFERENCES

Bernstein, B. (1993, June). *Ethical issues.* Presented at *Psychotherapy Finances* Managed Care Conference.

Case manager qualifications in AMBHA member companies (1996, Apr.). Washington, DC: American Managed Behavioral Healthcare Association.

The continuum of ambulatory behavioral healthcare services (1995). Alexandria, VA: Association for Behavioral Healthcare.

Contracting decisions based on outcomes data (1995, Mar.). Tallahassee, FL: Mental Health Corporations of America.

Defino, T. (1996). Behavioral health management: Carve-out, carve-in, and fully integrated models. (CSCSW clinical update.) *Health System Leader*, Oct. 2(8), 4–11.

Donahue, M. & Wirecki, M. T. (1995). Knowing What Insurers Want. *The Complete Capitation Handbook* (p. 67). Tiburon, CA: Jossey-Bass.

Gruttadarro, D. (1996, Feb.). *AMBHA's national behavioral credentialing verification service.* Presented at Global Business Research Ltd.'s conference on Behavioral Healthcare Provider Profiling.

Harris, Scott (1991, Dec.). Treatment planning: A managed care guide to the rules of the road. *CPA Briefings: Managed Care*, No. 107.

Montgomery, J. S. (1995, May). *Advances in provider credentialing and recredentialing.* Presented at Institute for Behavioral Healthcare's Conference on How to Improve and Customize Behavioral Healthcare Provider Networks.

Rovner, J. (1995). Credentialing HMO physicians. *HMO*, Nov./Dec., 60–63, 66–68.

Sabin, J. (1995). Developing and marketing time-limited therapy groups. *Psychiatric Services Journal, 46*(1), 7–8.

Tuttle, G. (1995). Industry analysis: A look at managed behavioral care. *Practice Strategies, 1*(7), 1–4.

Tuttle, G. (1996). Guess who's coming to lunch: New industry standards mean managed care visits to provider offices. *Practice Strategies, 2*(3), 5–6.

3

The Shapes We're In

> The decision to affiliate with another professional cannot be predicated only on mutual liking.
>
> *Robert Henley Woody, Ph.D., J.D.*

By and large, psychotherapists practiced as loners for many years, valuing and enjoying their autonomy. Smaller practices handled their own scheduling and billing, with little overhead other than office rent, furniture, and a sound muffler.

The earliest ventures into group practice were on the West Coast in the late 1980s and early 1990s, as providers with common clinical values and concerns about increasing managed care requirements met informally for peer review and case management.

The list of managed care demands grew longer: central intake, triage, quality assurance, outcomes management, patient satisfaction, electronic claims filing capability, multiple office sites, and multidisciplinary staffs to handle diverse caseloads. Informal peer review groups decided to sell their services under one name, applying to managed care panels as "groups without walls," and listed their individual practices as multiple sites to trigger referrals by zip codes.

Managed care firms asked for greater accountability from the group practices, whose members were looking for new ways to meet malpractice insurance requirements, share expenses, and provide backup for 24-hour coverage. Many groups were beginning to consider "at-risk" financial arrangements, including capitation and case rate pricing. Both require legal structures that can assume liability and accept risk.

Entrepreneurial clinicians are leaders of the new multidisciplinary, multispecialty practices of dozens of therapists in staff models with their own networks of providers. Those practices have become mini-managed-care carve-outs, or preferred provider organizations (PPOs).

Other popular group entities include independent practice associations (IPAs), provider hospital organizations (PHOs), management services organizations (MSOs), and traditional structured group practices. Some groups of providers have made significant investments in designing, or buying and implementing, sophisticated practice models, only to find that their best efforts cannot keep pace with market demands for technology and capital. (See Exhibit 3.1).

A number have been sold to larger companies, or merged as behavioral health care departments of hospital delivery systems. Some group practices have simply unraveled their systems and are rebuilding to serve more diverse markets of third-party and private-pay clients. In some areas, managed care firms are informally bringing select providers together, designing their own groups without walls.

Clearly, the direction for providers at this time is to affiliate with at least one group entity in order to benefit from computerized data systems, tap volume referrals from group contracts, and market specialty services within a broad continuum of care. Depending on the maturity of local public and private managed care systems, it may be too late or too early for providers to form group practices.

In a developing market, it makes sense for providers to come together as a structure that can expand with its own network of independent contractors for the purpose of contracting with hospital-driven systems, and to act as a ready-made provider network for HMOs entering the market.

In a saturated market, providers might find it more prudent to look for linkages along a broad continuum of care, tapping the money stream at

EXHIBIT 3.1. Medical Services Integration.

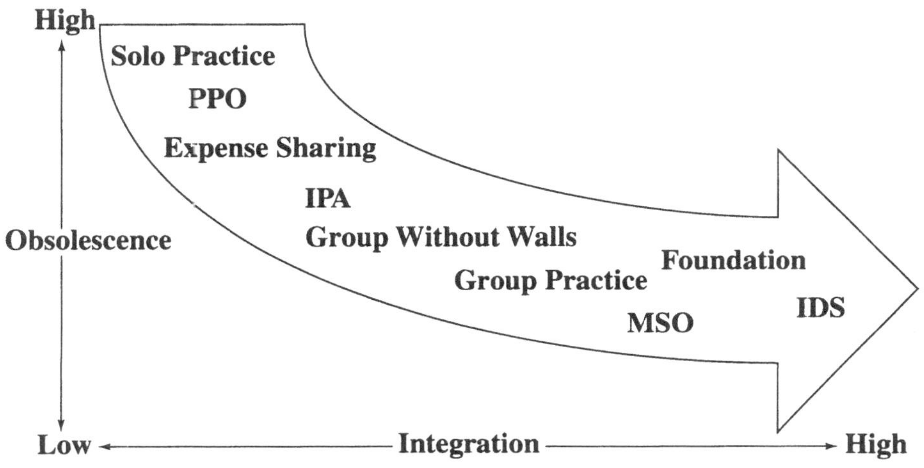

several points. Providing specialty services to a number of systems—including large group practices with carve-out and HMO contracts, hospital-driven systems, day treatment programs, EAPs, and regional networks of community mental health centers—allows clinicians to draw on the market clout of those systems, without substantial cash outlays.

There is no national boilerplate group practice model that guarantees success in every market. But providers who know what their local community is willing to purchase, and adjust clinical skills to meet those needs, will have the better chance.

FORMING A GROUP PRACTICE

Q What are the advantages of group practices?

A It takes less time for managed care firms and other payers to reach providers when they are in a group practice. It's easier for case managers to track client referrals. There also tends to be a greater sense of trust between the case managers and the providers in the group practice. Payers view groups as more experienced, with time-efficient treatment, ongoing peer review, administrative systems, and an understanding of the importance of the patient's benefit plan.

The group system is more responsive to the needs of the insurance/managed care industry. It has a level of complexity and sophistication that answers the needs of these organizations and their patient/clients. Often, preferred group practices develop special programs that support the needs of their client companies. (See Exhibit 3.2).

Q What are the characteristics of a preferred group practice?

A Preferred group practices share the following characteristics: problem-solving ability; rapid response capability; a clear definition of providers as a group practice, not as competing private practices; flexibility; and an interdisciplinary structure. Also, they offer multiple treatment formats (individual, group therapy, family therapy, after-care groups, multifamily groups); have a symptom-reduction psychotherapy orientation, with an understanding of intermittent care; and are results oriented.

EXHIBIT 3.2. Why Form a Group Practice?

Weak Reasons	Better Reasons
1. Security	1. Expanded continuum of care
2. To ride other providers' coattails	2. Economy of scale
3. Scared	3. To improve clinical quality
4. Less work, more money	4. To regain clinical autonomy
5. At least you're doing something	5. To accept at-risk contracts

Q Is it true that it costs several thousand dollars to start a group practice?

A The biggest expenses involved in forming a group structure capable of accepting capitated contracts are legal and accounting fees and management information system (MIS) investments. Add to those the consulting fees for developing practice guidelines and treatment protocol, credentialing systems, quality assurance programs, outcomes measurement tools, and marketing materials. Even groups that rely on provider investments of time and cash will spend more than $60,000. Some sell their guidelines, in binders and on computer disks that can be customized, for $3,000 to $5,000. For providers who are serious about starting a group practice, the templates can be a real bargain. Other providers who are looking for a cheap, quick fix are disappointed, because even with templates, they still face legal, accounting, and system fees, along with hard work.

Q What are the types of group practices?

A The structures most often used by behavioral health care providers are PPOs, IPAs, Groups Without Walls (GWW), traditional group practices, and MSOs. (See Exhibit 3.3.) Legal entities vary within the group structures. The most popular new legal structure is a limited liability company (LLC). Each state has its own laws and restrictions about what legal structure can be used for professional services. Check with an attorney who specializes in health care law early in the process of creating a group.

EXHIBIT 3.3. Group Structure Definitions.

PPO: An organization of independent providers who join to contract with managed care firms and offer discounted fees for service. Some or all of the participating providers usually own the network. The PPO contracts for the services, but the entity does not provide the services. It can be a business corporation or partnership, rather than a professional corporation. PPOs do not share economic risk.

IPA: Independent practitioners share the risk in managed care contracting under a stand-alone business entity—usually a professional corporation or partnership owned by the providers. At least 50% of shareholders and 51% of the equity must be held by one category of professionals. IPA members do not share overhead costs, and they can compete for non-IPA business. The structure can serve both as a PPO and as a provider delivery system under capitated contracts. It is often the structure of choice for regional alliances of several small to middle-sized group practices.

GWW: Providers remain in their own practices, but pool money for central intake, answering services, administrative services, insurance and other benefits and contracting with managed care firms. It's the most flexible arrangement for providers who want to remain in solo practices. At least 20 to 30% of income must be pooled under existing antitrust regulations to ensure that providers actually function as a group and are not meeting to fix prices. While some early GWWs have tightened to structured group practices, it remains a popular option in developing managed care markets. That's largely because the investment is limited and providers can pull out fairly easily.

Traditional Group Practices: This is a tight business structure, usually a staff model where providers are employed and share profits. They are usually owned by a single proprietor, partners, or a small group of investors. The group practice may act as an MSO for other providers, or develop its own network of providers for referrals.

MSO: A business structure designed to manage contracting, leasing, purchasing, billing, and computerized communications for a clinical practice. It allows nonclinicians to partner with clinicians. It's a popular system for regional networks competing for employer contracts. A number of large managed care firms offer MSO services to provider groups, often as a first step toward purchasing the practice.

PHO: Provider hospital organization. A joint venture between provider groups and hospitals or facilities where the hospital acts as the contracting agent for managed care business. The providers allow the facility to offer a broader continuum of services for one-stop shopping.

Q Where do I find a lawyer who specializes in health care law?

A Many state bar associations have directories of members who concentrate on health care law. The American Bar Association (312-988-5580) has a health law division and will provide names of members in your area. The National Health Lawyers Association (202-833-1100) is another good resource. If those resources fail, try asking the attorney for a local hospital or psychiatric facility for a referral. Also, attorneys who have handled cases before the state licensing boards are likely to have health care contracting experience.

Q What are the basics of forming a group practice?

A Requirements for various group structures vary. But consultants working with providers to develop or change group practices suggest these basic steps for any structure (Tuttle, 1995).

1. ***Develop a mission statement.*** What is the purpose of the group, and what services will it provide? (See example in Exhibit 3.4.)
2. ***Decide which group structure and legal entity match the purposes set forth in the mission statement.*** This is the time to outline a business plan. An attorney and an accountant should be part of the process.
3. ***Design the group's clinical protocol and treatment guidelines.*** This is a standard set of operating guidelines that tells purchasers and clients how they can expect the group consistently to provide services.
4. ***Design a system for quality assurance and outcomes measurement.*** It should be an extension of the treatment guidelines and clinical protocol, and a step toward marketing.
5. ***Create a plan for marketing*** the group's services to private-pay, managed care, public-sector, and employer customers.

Q Why are managed care companies shifting to work with group practices?

EXHIBIT 3.4. Statement of Purpose and Goals.

Access Behavioral Care is a multidisciplinary, fully integrated behavioral health specialty group.

ABC's goals are:

1. To provide a broad range of cost-effective, high-quality mental health services to the community, including wellness and preventative care strategies.
2. To implement strategic planning to adapt successfully as a group and as individuals to the constantly changing environment of behavioral health care.
3. To contract as a group with managed care companies, health plan, and medical groups on a fee-for-service and/or shared-risk basis.
4. To create strategic alliances with health care entities to maximize services and infrastructure, and to successfully compete in the marketplace.

Source: Access Behavioral Care, Inc. Los Angeles, CA. All rights reserved by Access Behavioral Care, Inc. Reprinted with permission.

A It's easier, more efficient, and less expensive. The reward for the group practices is more clinical autonomy and more referrals. On the down side, the group practices are expected to take on an incredible amount of responsibility for patient care, and administrative and quality tasks.

Managed care firms spend up to 17% of the benefit dollar assigned to behavioral health on monitoring and supervising network providers. The companies realize a savings when they can make a single call to a group practice for one-stop shopping—especially when that group already follows similar clinical guidelines. Other efficiencies that attract managed care firms to group practices include centralized billing, enhanced computer systems, multiple specialties, physician availability for medication management, ability to handle crises, and office staff trained to communicate effectively with the managed care staff.

There is a question of relative success for the provider group in this case. Frustrated practice owners report that clinicians are working faster and harder to serve an increased number of clients, and handle new reporting and quality assurance responsibilities for lower fees. In fact, several of the most sophisticated and efficient group practices have been sold to managed care firms because they couldn't keep pace with industry changes.

Q What are some of the most important issues to consider when starting a group practice?

A What is your purpose in forming a group practice? What can you achieve through a group practice that can't be accomplished in a solo practice? The most likely reasons to form a group are to create a one-stop shopping setting for contracting with managed care payers, and to achieve savings through economies of scale. Creating a group is by no means an instant solution to practice problems. In fact, it will raise a number of new issues. How are you selecting your partners? Agreement on clinical philosophy is important, but balancing clinical skills with business and marketing skills is a better way to ensure stability. Many consultants who help providers form group practices suggest a weekend retreat where some of the worst-case market and clinical scenarios are played out. It's also a good time for providers to develop a group mission statement—the basis for selecting a legal structure and developing a business plan, clinical protocol, and marketing plan. Including an attorney and an accountant for some part of the retreat is a good idea.

Key issues include legal and tax considerations; equity and capitalization; governance and control; credentialing and clinical fit; shared risk, investments, and compensation; and non-competition issues.

Q What are the basic steps to take in order to be in business once we decide to start a group?

A The basics are as follows: conduct a name search, get a business license and a taxpayer identification number, incorporate legally, adjust malpractice coverage, and set up a bank account.

Q Operationally, what do I have to do to start a group?

A Initially, you have to complete your business plan, estimate realistically the number of current clients being seen by members of the practice, and anticipate the volume of new members. Based on these projections, the following operational issues need to be addressed: deciding on office space and number of clinical sites, estimating equipment and supply needs, acquiring marketing materials, recruiting staff, hiring an accountant, hiring a health care attorney, and setting up a system for provider credentialing.

Q What are some of the policies that need to be in place before the group practice starts operation?

A Group practices' shareholders and affiliates need to operate according to the same policies. To accomplish this, the policies must be in writing and signed by all group practice participants. To decrease the amount of risk exposure for the legal business entity, the following specifications should be established: quality assurance, risk management, confidentiality, eligibility verification, reporting and audit requirements as requested by the accountant, referral obligations, and care approval mechanisms (Zieman, 1993).

Q Are there contractual obligations that shareholders and providers should agree to before officially joining the group?

A It is important that members of the group have contractual obligations to one another. Thus, it is also important that all of the following issues be fully discussed and outlined in a memorandum of understanding that each participant in the group practice signs. Robert Henley Woody (1989), an attorney who works with mental health providers, suggests the following.

- Financial duties: What will each member pay initially and monthly? If there is a financial loss, for what percentage is the provider responsible? Will majority shareholders be required to submit financial statements?
- Rights and obligations: What are the rights and responsibilities of providers and shareholders in terms of reconciliation of bank and financial accounts, legal actions, decision making, selection of new associates, and termination (voluntary and involuntary), and how will tangible and intangible assets be figured?
- Compensation: Who sets fees? Will everyone be charging the same fees? How will money be collected and distributed?

- Noncompetition: If a provider leaves the group, may he or she take managed care contracts, or do they stay with the group practice? Will providers be allowed to operate private practices or to work for other groups that might run competing programs?
- Trade secrets: What about restricting access to client names, mailing lists, group practice forms, outcomes, or patient satisfaction surveys?
- Termination decisions: Who has the authority to fire a provider? What if the provider doesn't pay his or her monthly share of expenses during startup? Is there a buy/sell agreement?

How liable am I for other clinicians in a rent-sharing group?

If the clinicians represent themselves as a group on a letterhead or in any type of advertising, marketing, or contracting listing, there is assumed liability, according to most health care attorneys. That includes sharing a Yellow Pages advertisement listing in the telephone book. Some attorneys suggest using a practice name to register a DBA (doing business as) with the local county government. They also recommend that practice members coordinate their malpractice coverage through the same carrier to address shared liability issues. The bottom line is how the group would be perceived by a court. Most courts have viewed liability from the perspective of the client and how the clinicians have represented themselves in advertising. Keep in mind that clinicians are responsible if they know that someone is doing something wrong and then fail to act to correct the problem.

What must a group practice do to achieve success?

Lack of direction and lack of focus threaten any businesses entity. It is important that a group practice:

- Monitor finances diligently. How much is it bringing in daily, weekly, monthly? Track managed care payments by plans and diagnosis. Hire an accountant with health care experience.
- Know what it costs to provide services and make sure that the pricing structure allows a profit margin.

- Monitor referral services. Who's sending the business, or why isn't the group getting referrals?
- Develop a contract manual that covers all managed care agreements, fee structures, and compliance standards. Use it.
- Develop a practice policy manual that addresses those managed care requirements. Use it.
- Collect claims aggressively. Don't let payments drag beyond 30 days. Use electronic billing services for overnight postings and immediate collections.
- Avoid increases in overhead without increased income.
- Provide the specialized services that its customers want.

Q Is there special malpractice insurance to cover group practices?

A Most carriers endorsed by the major professional associations now offer a special group practice package, or they will work with groups to customize coverage to address the new practice issues. It is also important for group practices to insure their directors and officers. Those policies cover possible errors or omissions on the part of officers and directors in making business decisions that could affect clinical delivery. They do not cover malpractice, so clinicians serving on group practice boards should have both types of coverage.

Q What are the advantages and disadvantages of a staff model?

A For managed care firms, the key advantage of a staff model is the ability to control costs. Managed care firms use staff models where the pool of lives covered is large enough to support the hiring of several psychiatrists and social workers to operate from a clinic. Some managed care firms rotate providers from select group practices as rotating clinic staff on a part-time basis.

In those cases, the clinic staff is also the provider network, creating an interesting mix of questions concerning patient and employer responsibility.

Saul Feldman, CEO at U.S. Behavioral Health (now part of United Behavioral Systems), has advocated for provider networks, suggesting that the staff model loses the checks and balances that individual providers can bring to managed care as client advocates.

Although staff models help hold down managed care costs (one California firm trimmed its 100-member panel to 12 clinicians for a geographic area by switching to a staff model), the clinics often lack the flexibility and access that managed care companies demand of network providers. Clients wait longer for nonemergency appointments and generalists are usually favored over specialists, limiting access to certain therapy models.

Some provider groups that moved to staff models have suffered unanticipated increases in overhead as they took on the employer's shares of taxes, workers' compensation, and unemployment insurance. A number of those groups—especially practices that acted ahead of local market development—are scaling back, or returning to sole proprietorship with independent contractor networks.

Q What about MSOs? Is this a better way to work with managed care?

A A management services organization (MSO) is an entity created to provide business management, administrative, and contracting services for a group of providers. The owners of an MSO can also be owners of the clinical practice. The entity allows a clinician to partner with a nonclinician, usually someone with business expertise. Some managed care firms offer MSO services to group practices for a percentage of the profits. Others will pinpoint small practices, not quite up to snuff for a purchase, but worth enough investment to find out if the firm can help the group grow. The agreement would then allow the managed care firm to buy the practice, if the plan worked. MSO services can include renting office space, providing computer services, and contracting with managed care firms on behalf of the group.

There also are group practices that provide MSO services for individual providers. Separating clinical services from business functions works better for many providers, giving them some distance between the patient and their pocketbooks.

Q What if I'm in a group practice and I want out?

A Hopefully, you considered that when forming the group by including a buy/sell agreement, a legal document spelling out the terms of ownership when a partner wants to leave or is unhappy with the arrangement. If you did not, see an attorney before you take any steps.

GROUP OPERATIONS

Q What about group applications?

A Initially, all providers were required to apply to managed care firms as individuals. Then, about four years ago, the firms started to accept group applications as part of the trend toward partnering with select practices. Now, most managed care firms will accept group applications, but they insist on credentialing individuals within that group. In other words, not all individuals within a select group are guaranteed credentialing by a partner-managed care firm. This is in response to lawsuits based on sloppy credentialing and to national accreditation requirements.

Q What do group practices have to do in terms of credentialing providers?

A Group practices must meet many of the same credentialing standards as managed health care firms when they are assuming contracting liability for employees or independent contractors in a referral network. In fact, managed care firms attempt to cut costs by shifting as many credentialing tasks as possible to groups. Group practices should have written policies for credentialing—including primary-source verification—and recredentialing, investigating complaints against providers, selecting and terminating providers, and establishing requirements for participation in outcomes measurement and quality assurance programs.

Q How much overhead should a group practice expect to pay?

A A number of administrators of large group practices have suggested that overhead should not exceed 20% of revenue in the practice's budget. The Institute for Behavioral Healthcare's 1994 Council of Behavioral Group Practices Benchmarking Study found that administrative costs increased with group practice size, peaking at about 20 full-time clinicians. As groups grew past that point, the administrative costs decreased in proportion to the increase in clinical staff (Daniels, Kramer, & Mahesh, 1994).

Q **What should a group look for in a management information or computer system?**

A The data items needed in a group practice working with managed care include some or all of the following: enrollment, provider profiling, financial reporting, concurrent review, claim adjudication, preauthorization, co-payments, coordination of benefits, benefit verification, utilization, scheduling, outcomes measurement by diagnosis and clinician, and cost analysis.

Q **How is a customer-service-oriented group different from any other practice?**

A The characteristics of a customer-service-oriented group practice are that it has identified a number of customers, including the patient, the managed care firm, the employer, and the EAP; the providers hold themselves accountable for what happens to the patient; and they practice symptom focused therapy and are comfortable working with managed care firms.

Q **What are the most frequent customer service complaints about provider groups?**

A Customer service is the ability to provide service in such a manner that the customer is satisfied with the quality of the care.

Interestingly, most customers do not complain about the quality of the clinical interaction. What they do complain about is being left on hold, cold or rude reception by the office and staff, messy offices, dirty restrooms, failure to return routine calls, lack of information about patient insurance coverage or managed care benefits, long waits, the use of therapy time to complete paperwork, or the routine rescheduling of appointments.

SELLING A PSYCHOTHERAPY PRACTICE

Q When should a practice consider selling to a managed care firm?

A Providers usually start to consider selling their practices when they want to expand, but don't have the money; in order to take advantage of established marketing, contracting, and management information systems; or to attain economies of scale when overhead demands are outpacing income and investments.

Here are a few general benchmarks for established practices thinking of selling:

1. Practice has established 6 to 12 managed care/insurance contracts, two to three of them capitated. Purchasers look for demonstrated success in contracting in order to capture covered lives in a given area.
2. It has a profit margin of at least 4% to 6%. Expect to submit to standard audits and due diligence.
3. It is legally structured in a way that allows the transaction to occur smoothly.

See Exhibit 3.5 for a humorous view of the question.

Q Who will buy a mental health practice?

A Depending on the market and location, insurance companies, managed care companies, practice management firms, medical/surgical and psychiatric hospital systems, and behavioral and medical group prac-

EXHIBIT 3.5.

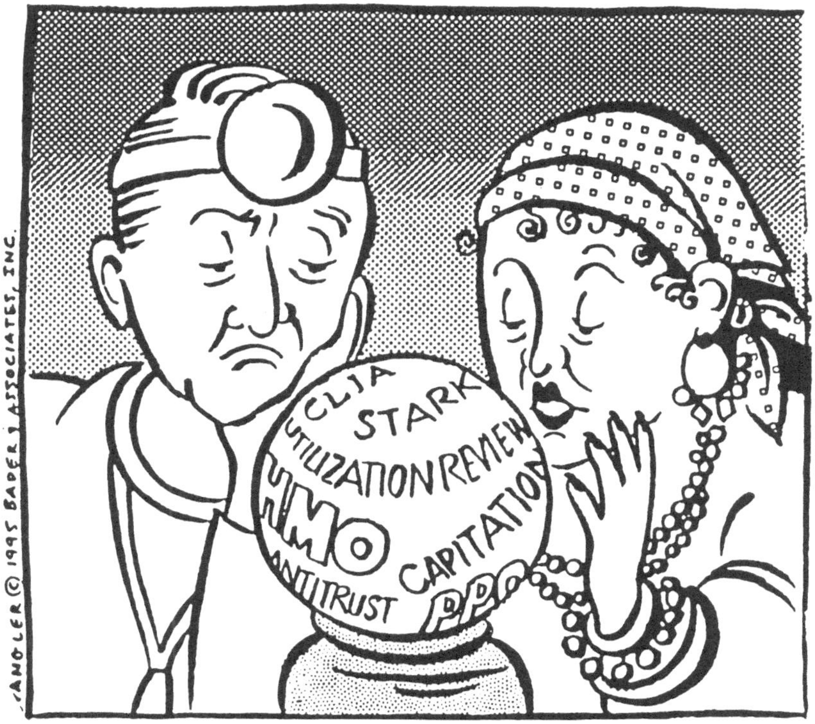

"I see this as a good time to sell your practice."

Source: Health System Leader. Courtesy of Capitol Publications, Alexandria, VA.

tices will buy a mental practice. Leading the pack are Apogee, Inc., Group Practice Affiliates, Merit's Continuum, and CMG Health, Inc.

Q Why do managed care firms want to own group practices?

A Behavioral health carve-out firms are searching for ways to remain players in a very fluid market. For some, that means becoming keepers of data. Other practices will be purchased by insurance companies. But most have realized that providers are critical to their success, and in many areas, the providers are becoming competitive with the carve-out firms. In order to stay in the chain, carve-out firms are stretching to become deliverers of care, and the easiest way to do that, and to reduce administrative overhead, is by owning the provider groups. The carve-out firm, in essence, becomes a provider system.

Q How much will buyers pay for a group practice?

A It hasn't been long since the value of a psychotherapy practice hinged mostly on the goodwill of the provider in his or her community. There was little equipment, other than office furniture. And there were very few actual recorded sales. Since 1992, the sales of practices have been booming. The most common purchase structures are straight-out purchases, joint ventures with options to buy, and management agreements with options to buy. A number of consultants have started to specialize as brokers for practices. One of the best in the business is Stan Grice at Advantage Marketing in Alexandria, Va. While there are any number of formulas for putting a pricetag on a practice, Grice has agreed to share one of the most common. (See Exhibit 3.6.)

Q So, do the buyers pay and the sellers can walk away?

A No. Buyers are still interested in the provider's goodwill. We do not know of any sales that do not involve the clinician's remaining for at least a transitional period. In most cases, the buyer expects the seller to remain an integral part of the practice group. That's why most buyouts in-

EXHIBIT 3.6. Sample Valuation Method.

1995	**Gross Revenue**
less	**Owner's Take = Earnings**
1995	**Earnings**
less	Salary to be paid to Seller
=	**Adjusted Net Earnings**
x	Multiple of x times adjusted net earnings (range is 4–6 times)
=	**Purchase Price**

Source: Sam Grice, Advantage Marketing, Alexandria, VA.

clude golden handcuffs, or delayed rewards based on future productivity and earnings. (See Exhibit 3.7.)

EXHIBIT 3.7. Sample Pay-Out Model.

- Purchase price is divided into portions, with an up-front cash payment to seller at closing and the rest rolled into an earn-out matrix.
- The earn-out is usually divided into three annual payments.
- Target gross revenue and net profit numbers are set for the next three years, and figured with the earn-out matrix.
- If the provider/seller exceeds the target numbers, earn-out payments will increase by a multiplier. Earn-out payments can be penalized if the targets aren't met.

Source: Sam Grice, Advantage Marketing, Alexandria, VA.

REFERENCES

Daniels, A. S., Kramer, T. L., & Mahesh, N. (1994). *Institute for Behavioral Healthcare, Council of Behavioral Group Practices, benchmarking study.* Portola Valley, CA: Institute for Behavioral Healthcare.

Tuttle, G. (1995, Dec.). *The many faces of group practices.* Presented to the South Carolina Association for Marriage and Family Therapy, Charleston.

Woody, R.H. (1989). *Business success in mental health practice.*

Zieman, G. (1993). Information systems and capitation contracting: Basic specifications for group practices. *Behavioral Healthcare Tomorrow, 2*(1), 40–43.

4

The Check Is in the Mail

They don't call it risk for nothing.

Monica Oss, Editor, Open Minds

Money is at the heart of all clinician complaints about managed care. There would be no utilization review, no treatment plans, no authorization for sessions—and no managed care firms, if money were not an issue.

Managed behavioral health care became an industry as a response to employer resistance to rising health care costs. True, there was a misperception that mental health and substance abuse were taking a disproportionate share of the benefit dollar. But the fact that psychotherapists had not set standards for measuring and documenting the effectiveness of their treatment, and for valuing their services, opened the door to third-party oversight.

Money remains the basis of all relationships between clinicians and managed care firms. That's because managed care firms are hired guns for employers. The role of the companies is to manage the employer benefit. All teamwork, partnering, and clinical quality issues aside, what clinicians want from managed care is a paycheck.

HOW DO I GET PAID?

Q How does managed care justify the choice of master's-level providers over psychologists and psychiatrists on the basis of fees alone?

A Managed care fee schedules usually vary by regions and are set by the companies' local or state directors. There are exceptions: U.S. Behavioral Health (now part of United Behavioral Systems), for example, has used one national fee schedule that doesn't vary with geographic markets. In either case, medical directors tend to look at fee schedules in terms of supply and demand. They study the market and note that psychiatrists historically have been paid more for their services. In addition, they are aware that psychiatrists are harder to recruit than are providers of other disciplines. And, given the higher level of risk associated with medication management and inpatient hospitalization, psychiatrists are paid a higher rate for those services.

While psychiatrists are paid a somewhat higher rate for psychotherapy services, many MDs who like to provide psychotherapy say they're missing out on referrals made to other clinicians who will take lower fees. That has prompted a call for universal, or flat, rates.

Psychologists have been paid more than master's-level clinicians based on the post-bachelor years required to gain a psychology degree and the supervised internships required for licensure. Companies tend to pay licensed clinical psychologists approximately $10 more per session.

Social workers and marriage and family therapists have typically received less than psychiatrists and psychologists. However, because the range of these disciplines allows the managed care companies the opportunity to pay a lower fee for the same quality of care for most mental health issues, they are often preferred by the companies and receive more referrals.

We see some companies flattening rates with a single fee for therapy and a different rate for medication management and inpatient management. In those settings, any provider of psychotherapy services is paid at the same $50, $60, or $70 rate.

The great equalizer is the case rate system. In this system, all providers (with the exception of medication management and inpatient hospitalization) are offered the same bundled rate. An example would be $500 for 1 to 12 sessions. The average national range is $200 to $400 for one year of outpatient treatment.

Under the case rate system, the psychiatrist, psychologist, marriage and family therapist, social worker, or licensed professional counselor is paid the same case rate and allowed to provide services that he or she considers clinically necessary.

Q How much do managed care firms pay?

A Fees vary by provider discipline, service provided, and geographic location. Providers can usually demand higher fees by moving to undeveloped markets, while the lowest fees will be paid in urban areas with competitive therapist markets. While most managed care fees fall within a predictable range, market demand can play to a provider's favor in convincing the companies to pay higher rates for a needed service that no one else offers. For example, most managed care firms will pay premium rates for therapists who are willing to be on 24-hour call for emergency room intervention and triage to prevent hospital admission.

The median fee paid for a 50-minute session of psychotherapy was $65, reports *Practice Strategies* in its 1996 managed care industry survey. That's a $10 decrease from 1995 median fees. Broken down by clinician license, the average fees reported in 1996 for a 50-minute individual session were $100.00 for psychiatrists, $68 for psychologists, and $59.00 for master's-level therapists, social workers, marriage and family therapists, and licensed professional counselors (Tuttle, 1995a 1996b). Fees for group therapy ranged from $30 to $64. And the 15 largest managed care firms responding to the survey reported paying a median fee of $86 for medical reviews by psychiatrists. Informally, therapists have reported managed care fees of as low as $30 for individual sessions.

Q Is a flat rate the same as a universal rate? What are the chances for universal rates?

A A universal rate would apply to psychotherapy rates, and then only under reduced-fees-for-services contracts. Since the market is shifting toward case rates and capitation, universal rates are not a major issue. While universal rates have been discussed by several large managed care firms, no company is taking steps toward adding a flat payment structure that would cross discipline lines. Psychiatrists who built practices based on psychotherapy say they aren't receiving psychotherapy referrals from managed care firms. Instead they are receiving referrals for medication management and sicker patients. They say that happens because it's cheaper for managed care to refer psychotherapy patients to other providers who charge less. Non-psychiatrists who have supported universal rates think it might raise their fees, but that's unlikely since most managed care reduced-fee rates are actually dropping.

Q I was offered $30 for a 45-minute session and asked to take evening hours. I agreed to the rate for day hours only, and the company told me to forget it, as there were

three other people who would take it. How can I make a living?

A Can you make a living at $30 for a 45-minute session? Three key factors will give you the answer. Does your practice mix include higher-paying work that will balance those referrals? Do you expect enough referrals under the arrangement to make it worthwhile? Do you know the cost to your practice of delivering a 45-minute session?

It is critical for providers to know the cost of business. When looking at your expenses, be sure to include these items: advertising/marketing; pagers; bookkeeping; dues and subscriptions; equipment leasing; malpractice insurance; office insurance; life, health, and disability insurance; license fees; payroll taxes; postage; professional fees; travel expenses; receptionist/secretary salaries; rent; pay-down salary; and costs at seminars, suppliers, telephone, utilities, office cleaning, and consultants.

If it costs the practice $25 to $30 to provide a 45-minute session and you don't have enough other work at higher fees to offset the lower fee, it won't work. Providers get ahead of the game by knowing their costs and the absolute bottom fee they will accept before negotiating contracts. For example, a provider might set $35 as a minimum fee if the cost of service is $25 and the provider needs a minimum clear profit of $10 per session.

Other providers who can accept the lower fees are saying (1) that their costs to provide services are lower than your cost to provide service, or (2) that they are accepting what is called the loss leader—that is, they are willing to lose money in order to get the business.

Q Blue Cross/Blue Shield of Colorado has shifted to a managed care approach for state employees. As a master's-level clinician, I have to pay an M.D. for supervision. At $45 per session, I can't afford supervision. I'm stuck. I have to be on the panel, yet I can't afford it.

A It is a tough position. One possible option would be to align with a group practice that includes a psychiatrist who signs off for the group practice. Another option is to compete for the Blues' patients by lowering your out-of-pocket fee to $45 for direct-pay clients.

Q Under what circumstances can a managed care firm deny payment for authorized provider services?

A If the contract specifies a time limit for submitting claims, the company can deny payment. One example is a managed care firm that requires providers to submit all claims within 60 days of each date of service. It clearly states that there is no obligation to pay if claims are received past that deadline. Some companies require that claims be filed within 60 days from the last date of service. Read your contracts carefully.

Some companies attach a window of opportunity to their authorizations, usually of 90 to 120 days. If the treatment is not provided before the expiration date, the company may not pay for the sessions. If the patient's coverage has lapsed, the company does not have to pay.

Q Can managed care companies pay for treatment and then demand that the money be returned?

A Yes. That's called retroactive deletion. A managed care firm might authorize treatment for a patient without knowing that the patient no longer is covered under an employer benefit plan. There's about a 30-day lag between the time employees are dropped from benefit plans and the time that information is entered into a data system. Providers are responsible for verifying patient coverage. In those cases, a company can deny coverage and demand repayment. Some providers negotiate managed care contracts to include clauses that would protect them from retroactive denials if treatment is authorized and the provider files complete treatment plans on time.

Q If the managed care company makes a mistake and authorizes treatment for a patient who isn't covered, who's responsible for payment?

A The patient. Most authorizations for treatment include a disclaimer, saying that if the patient isn't eligible, the company won't pay. Benefit information runs about 30 days behind, creating the opportunity for mistakes to be made. The provider would be responsible for collecting payment from the patient.

Q What if the managed care firm pays me too much? Do I have to return the extra fees?

A Yes. Most contracts also say that the company can hold the overpayments out of future payments.

Q **What does accepting assignment mean?**

A It means that the provider is agreeing to bill the insurer or managed care company directly for payment, asking the patient only for the co-payment. Providers who do not accept assignment collect from the patient and may or may not file the claim for the patient.

Q **If a company authorizes sessions for a patient with me, can I get paid if someone else in my practice sees that patient?**

A Probably not. Authorizations under fee-for-service plans and some case rates plans are specific to the provider's filing the treatment plan. The expectation is that he or she will be the treating provider. However, capitation plans allow more flexibility, with the provider group responsible for treatment decisions, as long as they meet contract requirements. Even in capitated agreements, some companies specify provider criteria.

Q **Can I bill managed care firms for missed appointments?**

A Missed appointments are the patient's responsibility and providers must collect payments from the patient. Most managed care firms accept practice policies for handling missed appointments, if those policies are in writing and are read and signed by the patient as part of the intake procedure. Managed care contracts usually address the issue, and some will place restrictions on how providers handle their referrals. For example, a patient may be allowed to miss one or two group sessions within a certain time without being penalized. Missed appointments should be documented in progress notes, however, because they can reflect on provider treatment outcomes.

Q **Can I bill the managed care company for time spent on paperwork?**

A Early in the development of managed behavioral health care, there were reports of angry providers who dashed off invoices for paperwork and telephone time. We don't know of any companies that paid the bills. Be careful what you sign. Agreements with managed care firms describe the procedures for filing treatment plans, requesting authorization for sessions, and billing. If you agree to provide the service for the offered fee, that's the deal. Streamlining the process by filing forms and claims electronically can cut down on time and costs.

AT RISK

Q **Please explain more about case rates. I've heard of case rates of $300 to treat a patient for an entire year. Does that mean six sessions?**

A Case rates really started to take hold for behavioral health services early in 1995. PacifiCare Behavioral Health began paying a select number of its provider groups a flat rate of between $250 and $450 to treat a patient for one year (Tuttle, 1995b). Rates varied with location and employer benefit plans. In this situation, groups are allowed to collect and keep copayments made by patients in addition to the case rate. Then it's up to the provider group to determine the level of services—individual therapy, group therapy, intensive outpatient therapy, or a combination—and which clinicians will provide the care. PacifiCare also pays a $1,000 case rate to select providers for crisis intervention and hospital diversion, up to nine days.

Under case rates, the provider group is at risk, but not to the degree seen under capitated contracts. Another example of case rates is offered by Merit Behavioral Care Corporation where the provider group is paid a flat $200 per referral for one year of care (Tuttle, 1996a). In this particular case, the provider has been guaranteed at least 300 referrals. The company offers a safety net by allowing the provider to return high-risk substance abuse or severely ill patients to its staff model. Also, the company has agreed in this case to consider the patient a new referral if he or she presents with new symptoms at least 90 days after the first episode of care has been completed.

Q What are some things that providers need to consider before entering a capitated arrangement?

A Is the provider prepared to hire other people to deliver services? The group practice provider network is essential to the delivery of services. Credentialing providers who support the group's clinical philosophy and make hours available to take referrals quickly is very important. Groups must know how much it costs per day to operate the practice. A central intake staff is needed, as well as financial resources to carry the practice during peak utilization periods.

When contracting, one should negotiate for payment on the first day of the month rather than on the last day. Make sure that the covered population is defined in the contract agreement. Leave openings to renegotiate when the managed care firm adds new clients who might change the population makeup and utilization patterns.

Psychological and pharmacological services need to be integrated, with a psychiatrist as part of the group practice. The group should be able to access and deliver a full continuum of care to include inpatient, partial, and day treatment; crisis intervention; home, outpatient, and stepdown care; and community resources.

Q A hospital has asked my group practice for a capitated proposal to cover 100,000 lives under its HMO contract. What should we look at to avoid risks?

A While there are a number of examples for calculating capitated pricing, there is no single formula that works for every contract. (See examples of capitated contract formulas in Exhibits 4.1 and 4.2.) To help minimize risks:

1. ***Know the covered population.*** Are the potential patients blue-collar workers, adolescents, working parents? What sort of services are they most likely to need, and how likely are they to access services? For example, a higher rate of substance abuse treatment can be expected with a larger number of covered adolescents.
2. ***Know the history.*** Ask to see insurance claims for the last two years to learn about past utilization. Anticipate higher utilization in the second and third years as employees become aware of new services.

EXHIBIT 4.1. Sample Capitated Rate Proposal.

Group Practice Costs

Overhead	$104,880.00
Inpatient	137,345.00
Outpatient	416,625.00
Total =	$658.850.00

divided by 46,668 lives for 12 months =
$1.18 per member, per month (rounded up from 1.1764841)

I. INPATIENT UTILIZATION ASSUMPTION

25 inpatient days per 1,000 =	1,167.5	days
Average length of stay, range	7.5–9.2	days
MD visits 90% of days =	1,050	days
Total MD Visits =	**1,050**	**days**

173 initial visits @ $110.00	$19,030.00
871 follow-up visits @ $95.00	$83,745.00
Total MD inpt. costs =	**$102,345.00**

PhD visits
(PhD provides testing on 20% of total admits = 70 patients)

70 patients @ $500 average cost for psychological testing =	$35,000.00
MD Costs	$102,345.00
PhD Costs	$35,000.00

Total Inpatient MD and PhD costs $137,345.00

II. OUTPATIENT UTILIZATION ASSUMPTIONS

Annual Utilization Rate

2.17% per 1,000 patients = 1,011 patients

6 visits average per patient x 1,011 patients = 6,066 visits

Average Outpatient Cost per Visit
(weighted average)

Provider Type	Initial Visit Cost	Follow-up Visit	Average # of Visits	Average Cost	% of Total Visits	Subtotal
MD	$110.00	$75.00*	5	$82.00	25	$2,000
PhD**	$70.00	$70.00	6	$70.00	37.5	$2,625
LCSW MFCC	$60.00	$60.00	6	$60.00	37.5	$2,250

Average Cost per Visit $68.75

Total Outpatient Provider Costs = 6,060 visits x $68.75 = 417,037.00

* Follow-up visits by MD include 2 complete hourly follow-ups and 2 30-minute medication follow-ups at $95/hr. rate.
** Includes psychological testing.

III. INDIRECT COST ASSUMPTIONS

A. Staffing	**Monthly Costs**
Intake, 1 hour/day @ $50.00	$1083.00
MD—utilization review and meetings 2 hours/week @ $95.00	823.00
Ph.D—utilization review and meetings 4 hours/week @ $70.00	1,213.00
Contract Administrator 2 hours/week @ $50.00	433.00
*Office Manager, 2 hours/week @ $25.00	215.00
*1FTE (Reception, clerical, billing) @ $18.00	3,120.00
PhD for Quality Assurance, 1 hour/week @ $70.00	303.00

* Includes federal and state taxes/benefits

Total Staffing per month	**$7,190.00**
	x 12
Total Staffing per year	**$86,280.00**

B. Equipment, Supplies, and Rent **$18,600.00**

(Includes facility costs, telephone, computer tax, postage, and office supplies.)

Total Overhead Costs = $104,880.00

Source: Compiled by Barbara Moss Keller, LCSW. Executive Director, Midpeninsula Mental Health Group, Inc., Palo Alto and Mountain View, CA. Reprinted with permission.

EXHIBIT 4.2. Sample Capitation Formula.	
100,000 lives covered for outpatient mental health and substance abuse treatment	
Utilization Assumptions	
3.5% penetration	3,500 patients
Average number of visits	6.0 visits
Total psychotherapy visits	21,000 visits
Average number of medication visits	2.0 visits
Total medication visits	7,000 visits
Costs	
Psychotherapy ($58 x 21,000)	$1,218,000
Minus copay collected ($18 x 21,000)	378,000
Total psychotherapy costs	840,000
Medication ($49 x 7,000)	$343,000
Minus copay collected ($10 x 7,000)	70,000
Total medication costs	$273,000
Total outpatient costs	$1,113,000
Per-member, per-month cost is calculated by:	
Total outpatient costs	$1,113,000
+ overhead costs	432,000
+ consultation costs	30,000
Total	$1,575,000
Divide by 100,000 = $15.77 per member, then divide by 12 to get a per member, per month cost of $1.31. Capitation cost: $1.31 per member, per month.	

Source: Gayle Zieman, Ph.D. (1995). How to Determine the Right Capitation Rates. Mesa Mental Health. Reprinted with Permission.

3. ***Leave wiggle room.*** Set a utilization range and add a clause that allows annual renegotiation if visits top the range. A number of group practices that signed early capitated agreements lost money when they were locked into long-term contracts. Those with good managed care partnerships have been able to add a yearly review clause.
4. ***Understand the benefits clearly.*** What are you agreeing to cover under the capitated contract? Aim for stop-loss clauses that allow you to return high-risk patients to the hospital or the HMO's staff model.
5. ***Build in 10%*** for profit/contingency funding.

Q Are there other ways to protect my group in a capitated contract?

A One tip from experienced group practices is to write into the contract capitation rates that are specific to age groups and capitate on those groups of patients where you know your costs of providing care. For example, the group could split out adolescents between 14 and 21 years of age and price differently for that population than for geriatric populations.

Another trend, mentioned earlier, is to leave an out for renegotiating prices if the population changes dramatically. Define the degree of change that would bring your partner back to the table.

Also, remember that even when the contract ends, the group may be responsible for completing treatment in progress that could last three to six months, and should budget for that continued care.

Q What is stop-loss insurance?

A Stop-loss insurance is coverage that guarantees that the amount of losses under a capitation agreement will not exceed a set dollar limit. Medical practices and hospitals have been purchasing stop-loss insurance for several years, but it may be fairly new to the behavioral health care field. Several insurance carriers have started offering the coverage, making pricing more competitive. The idea is to protect the provider group's bottom line. It requires careful monitoring of capitated contracts to make sure that claims forms are submitted regularly. That means that providers should be careful to budget for added staff time when bidding on capitated contracts that will carry stop-loss coverage. Ask your malpractice coverage carrier for a referral to agents offering stop-loss policies (Kreig, 1995).

PRICING STRUCTURES

Q What does it mean in terms of a capitated contract when people say per member, per month?

A The rate that is paid in advance is a projected dollar amount for providing defined services under a benefits package to a covered population and is broken down to a per member, per month figure. For example, $3 per-member, per-month for behavioral health services for a pool of 100,000 covered lives would be $300,000 per month. The group estimates the number of people who would utilize services during any given month, the type of services they are entitled to under a benefits package, the services that are likely to be delivered, the average length of treatment for those services, and the cost to deliver care. If the care can be delivered for less than the per-member, per month amount, the group makes money. If the services exceed the budget, the group loses money.

Q What is the average per-member, per-month rate for mental health services?

A Group practice rates for managed behavioral health and substance abuse range from 85 cents per member, per month for outpatient psychotherapy to $2.50 for inpatient and outpatient treatment. When group practices are subcontracting for capitation with carve-out firms, the companies will continue to provide 800 lines, intake and referral services, quality assurance monitoring, claims review, and customer service. The managed care capitation rate ranges between $15 and $20 per member, per month.

In capitated contracts for public-sector clients, rates can range from $17 to $30 per member, per month, for a much broader continuum of services, including outpatient care, case management services, residential treatment, foster care, forensic patients, and, in some cases, child welfare.

Q How do you know the right rate to charge if you're unsure of the marketplace? It all seems like guesswork.

A Eliminating guesswork is the provider's task before entering a capitated contract. Again, try to see the claims paid for the previous year for the population. Look carefully at the makeup of the group to be covered, and consider how likely its members are to utilize services. Only capitate on those services where you know the cost of treatment. One way to reduce risk is by eliminating certain diagnoses or services. Murray Zucker, M.D., suggests that providers might consider excluding coverage of chronically ill patients, psychiatric testing, electroconvulsive therapy, and ambulance charges when defining services in the contract (Zucker, 1994). Negotiate a separate fee schedule for certain services, or set utilization levels that would trigger higher reimbursement rates.

Q What population has the highest rate of utilization?

A Working people between the ages of 25 and 65 have the highest utilization rate. Women access behavioral health services more often than do men.

Q How many covered lives do I need to figure a capitated rate?

A In figuring the rate, 100,000 is a good basis. Most large group practices recommend against capitated contracts covering fewer than 40,000 lives.

Q What should the profit margin be?

A A common rule of thumb is 10% for profit/risk. Remember that it goes either way—profit or loss—based on predicted and actual utilization by the covered population.

Q Will capitated agreements allow my practice to use providers who aren't licensed in my state?

A That depends on what you agree to in your contract. In general, managed care firms are stepping away from micromanagement when they move to capitation. One of the bonuses providers expect under capitation is regained clinical and practice autonomy. But many of the employers who contract with the managed care firms have specified in their benefits packages that only licensed providers, or those of a particular discipline or with a particular license, should be used. Often, that's a case of following standard benefit language and not being familiar with the scope of practice of other providers or the status of state licensure. Still, managed care firms are going to follow the benefits structure. Also, managed care firms have to be mindful of accreditation requirements for licensure.

Where provider groups or delivery systems are contracting directly with the employer, the provider has the opportunity to influence the employer in terms of credentialing criteria.

REFERENCES

Keller B. (1993, June). "Service Utilization Assumptions." Presented at Capitated Arrangements Workshop at the Psychotherapy Finances Managed Care Conference.

Kreig, J. (1995, May/June). Stemming the risk of capitated contracts: What providers should consider when buying stop-loss insurance. *Health Care Innovations*, pp. 12–16.

Tuttle, G. (1995a). Industry analysis: A look at managed behavioral health care. *Practice Strategies, 1*(7), 1–5.

Tuttle, G. (1995b). Industry trends: Numbers are in for one MCO that's using average billings to set case rates. *Practice Strategies, 1*(5), 4–5.

Tuttle, G. (1996a). Making case rates pay. *Practice Strategies, 2*(1), 1–7.

Tuttle, G. (1996b). An industry update: MCOs report lower fees, broader services. *Practices Strategies, 2*(8), 1–4.

Zieman, G. (1995, Feb.). "How to Determine the Right Capitation Rule." Presented at the Institute for Behavioral Health Conference on Advanced Behavioral Group Practice Management.

Zieman, G. (1995). *The Complete Capitation Handbook.* Philadelphia: Jossey-Bass.

Zucker, M. (1994, June). *How to form a group.* Presented at Psychotherapy Finances' Conference on Critical Provider Issues.

5

To Market, To Market

> The reality is that most good clinicians engage in marketing every day.
>
> *Jeri Davis,* President, Jeri Davis Marketing Consultants

Providers are reluctant to think of what they do as a business. "I haven't found a psychotherapist yet who isn't filing an income tax return reporting the money they make offering services," says Samuel Mayhugh, president of Behavioral Care Health Systems. "But many still don't want to think of their services as what produces their paychecks."

The solution for many good clinicians with weak business skills is to hire administrators or consultants to package, sell, and acquire contracts for their services. In some cases, practices buy those administrative services from managed care firms acting as management services organizations (MSOs). The Brick Kiln Provider Network, Inc., on Long Island, N.Y., is an example of a practice that separated marketing and administration from its clinical services by building a small MSO for contracting purposes.

Regardless of the structure that providers choose, the shift to business thinking is basic to success in a market where third-party payers, employers, and private-pay clients are being educated as consumers who shop for quality and value in behavioral health services.

While clinicians balk at the thought of marketing and accepting credit card payments, many who have tried to package and sell their services have found that they're really very good at it. That's so because they are naturals at listening. The key to all good marketing is listening, and hearing what the customer wants, rather than selling what you think the customer needs.

For managed behavioral health care providers, there is more than one customer. The first customer is the patient, the second is the managed care firm, and the third is the employer who pays for the service.

Often overlooked as a marketing target, the employer also holds the power to make final decisions on benefits packages. The employer determines which providers will be reimbursed and which services will be covered. Remember, the managed care firm's job is to administer the benefits plan selected by the employer, at a savings in cost whenever possible.

So, marketing to the employer means listening to learn what makes the company unique, and about the special needs of its employees. How can your clinical skills meet those employee needs? And can you measure your work in terms of the employee's ability to function?

If you can name that tune, you are halfway home when it comes to marketing to the managed care firm. Managed care firms are looking for providers who will work with them to help meet employer needs. Good companies don't forget that providers are their most important investment.

As for marketing to the patient, managed care firms use satisfaction surveys to ask patients about convenient hours, easy-to-reach locations, and safe, well-lit offices with plenty of parking space. Making quality providers available quickly, and offering a full range of services, assures steady managed care referrals.

GETTING IN

Q How many managed mental health care companies are there?

A There were as many as 400 such firms during the early 1980s, but the number has dropped considerably through industry mergers and acquisitions. Now, fewer than two dozen large national managed behavioral health care firms control the market share. That does not take into account, however, HMOs with behavioral health networks, regional and statewide managed behavioral health care firms, or companies specializing in partial hospitalization or day treatment, or that own or manage behavioral group practices. The larger mental health firms are listed in Appendix C.

Q How can I find out which companies are in my area and when or how to apply?

A Contact the national offices for the larger firms listed in Appendix C and request a provider application. Often the companies will ask which state you're calling from and refer you to a regional office for an application. If you're transferred to the provider relations department, ask if the company is doing business in your state.

For other companies, a good starting point is to call your state insurance commissioner's office and request a list of all managed care firms licensed to do business in the state, and also a list of those with license applications pending. Ask if the insurance commission has a managed care division, which will know of state or local trade associations for HMOs and other managed care firms. Other possibilities are to contact the local Chamber of Commerce and request a listing of all health plan members. Classified advertisements and display ads in local or state magazines will feature managed care plans marketing to employers.

Then it's simply a routine task of calling the companies, asking for their provider relations department, and requesting an application.

Q I've filled out several applications but never received a response. What do I do now?

A Don't give up. As you are mailing applications, or letters requesting applications, set up a tickle file to remind yourself to follow up with a telephone call in three to four weeks. If you're checking on an application, you may be told that there are no panel openings. If so, make another reminder to check back later. Companies regularly win new contracts or build businesses through mergers. Local provider relations managers need to know about therapists who are available. Companies don't send out applications as casually as they once did, primarily because of the cost involved in setting up credentialing files that include primary-source verification. So, if you receive an application, there's a good chance that the company needs you. If you don't hear within a reasonable time after you apply, call the provider relations department, starting with the regional office. One California counselor says that when she checked on an application, she learned that her acceptance letter had been mailed to Albany, N.Y., rather than to her in Albany, Calif.

Q I keep hearing about specialties. What is there left to specialize in?

A Specialize in what you're interested in and what you're trained to do well. While it is true that having the right specialty listed on your profile will draw referrals from case managers, your good fortune won't last long if you aren't truly a specialist in that area. Some managed care firms have developed criteria for identifying specialists to match diagnoses. Merit Behavioral Care Corporation, for example, has recruited an interim panel to test its plan for matching specialists to clinical treatment areas, including abuse, addictions, AIDS, biofeedback, child/adolescent problems, eating disorders, geriatrics, group therapy, and marital/family issues.

Other companies recognize certification or clinical membership in professional associations as designating specialist status. Most firms continue to look for child psychiatrists and providers who specialize in forensics, workers' compensation, and bicultural/bilingual issues. Ask case mangers with managed care firms about specialty needs. Then identify your top three clinical skills, keeping those needs in mind, and support them with documentation of training, experience, and any certification. Then talk to case managers with managed care firms to make sure that those specialities are shown in your profile.

Q I seem to spend a lot of time making pink and blue fliers and buying stamps. How do I know whether this works?

A You won't know until you start tracking new clients by referral sources. Include on the intake form a question that asks how the client learned about your practice or program. Identify a target audience for marketing rather than using a shotgun approach. Add coupons for discounts or free initial visits to promotional materials and code them for tracking. Nothing elaborate is required, but set up a file for each product line and keep track of postage, printing, faxes, and promotional events, and match those against your referrals after six months or a year. Target two or three products for promotion at any one time, staggering additional groups or specialities for marketing every few months. Look at your efforts and results at the end of each year to see what works before planning for the next year. Set reasonable goals for each product, or you will always be swimming against the current.

Q What are the best niche markets under managed care?

A The best niche market is a service that's needed, but is not already provided in your area by another clinician. Start with an inventory of your clinical skills. Ask managed care payers and employers what they need. Don't forget to list what your clients have requested, or referral needs that you've identified for your clients. Match the needs with your skills. Then package and price the services creatively.

Examples of Niche Markets

Eating disorders
Stepfamily programs
Workers' compensation programs
Gay and lesbian services
Chronic illnesses management (HIV, cardiac, asthma, cancer)
Adolescent programs with after-school transportation
Pain control
Geriatrics
Infertility/menopausal/PMS issues
Forensics
DUI sentencing alternatives
Bilingual/bicultural
Sign language
In-home care
Parenting
Weight control
Couples workshops
Corporate consulting
Plastic surgery
Sex therapy
Stress management
Wellness and preventive care
Codependency
Targeted services for racial and ethnic groups

Q **Do I need a consultant to help with marketing? If so, how do I find one, and how much should I pay?**

A The answer is determined by how aggressively you want to market your practice, how much money you have to spend, and whether you or other practice members have expertise in marketing and the time to make the contacts.

Marketing is a very general term that should draw on a business plan and a clear definition of the group's mission statement and to package clinical skills for sale to managed care firms, employers, facilities, and private-pay clients. A marketing plan should be based on an assessment of market needs, an analysis of what competitors are already providing (as well as the potential for those competitors to become allies, or even purchasers of your services) and an assessment of your group's capability to meet market needs. Assuming those steps have been taken, the group begins networking to sell services.

Practitioners often overlook business and industry contacts that can benefit the practice, but once directed, many do an excellent job of marketing and contracting. However, most have limited time and marketing falls to the bottom of a long list of tasks. Some groups designate one member as the marketing and contracting representative, who is paid for those services at the same level as other group members are paid to provide clinical services.

Managed care networking requires regular contacts and familiarity with market needs and pricing. Many group practices turn to consultants to take them from a business plan to contracts. Average hourly fees range from $100 to $150, with discounts for volume. The average daily fee for consultants working with group practices ranges from $1,000 to $1,500, plus expenses. Most will provide a proposal of up to two pages free, but groups should expect to pay for anything else (Martin & Tuttle, 1994).

Many consultants are clinicians who have learned the managed care ropes through their own practices. Others come to the field from marketing or managed care firms. Some who were eager to work with group practices a few years ago say they're less interested now, citing unrealistic provider expectations and slow payment from group practices. Exhibit 5.1 lists some tips for working with consultants. A checklist for interviewing consultants appears in Exhibit 5.2.

Q If I read in the business section of my newspaper that an employer has hired a managed care firm, what do I do next?

A Ask yourself some questions: What do I know about the employer? What are the special needs of a company that makes widgets? Are the workers under particular types of stress? What skills do I have, or what

EXHIBIT 5.1. Tips for Working with Consultants.

1. Set clear goals that meet the consultant's skills. Don't hire a consultant with national networking contacts if you are trying to develop local employer business.
2. Decide how much you have to spend and give the consultant a reasonable working budget.
3. Remember that knowledge and contacts are what consultants have to sell. Don't ask for free advice.
4. Expect consultants to provide a monthly report of contacts made, appointments scheduled, and proposals submitted.
5. Consider working with more than one consultant on a per-project basis. For example, product development is very different from pricing and contract negotiation.
6. Interview past clients. Ask if the consultant delivered the work on time.

Source: Karen Martin and Gayle M. Tuttle (1994). "Dos and Don'ts of Working with a Consultant." Presented at Psychotherapy Finances Second Annual Managed Care Conference.

services do I offer that seem to match that employer's needs? Write a letter of introduction (keep it brief) to the managed care firm's director of provider relations. Congratulate him or her on the new contract. Tell the company that your office is located within a 15-minute drive from the area in which many of the new client's employees live. Say enough about the employer to show the managed care firm that you know your community—and the client's. Mention services offered, hours, locations, access, and interest. Request an application.

Send a copy along with a cover letter to the human resources manager at the local employer. Congratulate the company on its choice of mental health firms. Mention that you have applied as a provider and hope to be able to serve, or continue to serve, its employees. (A sample letter of introduction is shown in Exhibit 5.3.)

Q What about group therapy?

A Group therapy has been gaining attention as provider groups have taken on large client populations under case rate and capitation contracts. The result is that clinicians are booking more client hours at lower

EXHIBIT 5.2. Consultant Interview Log.

Aspect	Cons. #1	Cons. #2	Cons. #3	Cons. #4	Comments
Telephone presence					
Interest in project					
Industry knowledge/ breadth of experience					
Experience with specific type of project					
Knowledge of local market					
Business philosophy					
Reference checks					
Fees/payment strategy (including travel)					
Customer service					
Reference checks Overall communication skills					
Motivation					
Industry/managed care contacts					
Affiliations with lawyers, accountants, etc.					
Availability					
Responsiveness					
(GUT LEVEL FEELING)					

Source: Karen Martin. Martin & Assoc., Santa Monica, CA. Reprinted with Permission.

EXHIBIT 5.3. Sample Letter of Introduction.

Please B. Kind, Director of Provider Relations
ABC Managed Care
101 Closed Panel Way
Anywhere, America 55555

Dear Ms. Please B. Kind,

Congratulations on ABC Managed Care's new contract to manage behavioral health care for Large Employer Widgets in MyTown. My group, Very Good Providers, Inc., has enjoyed a number of LEW employees as clients in the past.

Since our multidisciplinary group of 15 providers would like to continue to serve your new client, I am writing to tell you about Very Good Providers and to request both group and individual application forms.

Our multispecialty practice includes licensed psychiatrists, psychologists, clinical social workers, and marriage and family therapists who have treated adults, adolescents, children, and geriatric patients for 14 years. We offer medication management, individual and group therapy, intensive outpatient programs, and psychoeducational services, and rely on a strong network of self-help and support groups as referral resources, where appropriate.

Very Good Providers' clinicians offer services during extended evening and weekend hours at three sites, including a primary care physician's office. All are within an easy 30-minute drive of LEW. Routine appointments can be scheduled within three to five workdays, and our staff is available 24 hours each day for emergency and urgent care.

Enclosed is a summary of specialty services offered and a menu of therapy groups. I look forward to receiving ABC applications, and would enjoy an opportunity to share with you some of Very Good Providers' outcomes and patient satisfaction survey results. If Very Good Providers can be of assistance in the meantime, don't hesitate to call us at 800-555-5555.

Sincerely,

M.C. Friendly
Very Good Providers
Easy Access Street
MyTown, USA 66666

reimbursement rates—a losing combination. As managed care payers have encouraged providers to move toward less restrictive treatment settings, more group practices have started looking to group therapy as a way to provide cost-effective care.

The group described in the case rate example of 300 referrals at $200 each relies heavily on therapy groups with a length-of-treatment goal of 3.5 sessions for individuals in order to be profitable. Other group practices are setting goals of shifting 20% of their clients into therapy groups to relieve provider overload. Clinicians are rewarded with time off and bonuses when they create and run successful therapy groups.

Those practices have included a screening for potential group members as part of intake so that clients consider both individual and group therapy as a possibility during their assessment visits. Some clinicians have added measures to guard against overutilization of group therapy. One practice includes a checklist at intake to measure functionality, coping skills, previous therapy results, and client willingness to participate in a group. (Tuttle, 1996).

Group therapy is also popular with private-pay clients because it's more affordable. A key selling point is to use package pricing for a set number of sessions. Some practices package group therapy with individual sessions, for example, four group meetings of 90 minutes each with two one-hour individual sessions.

Managed care rates for group therapy allow a clinician to make more money than by seeing individuals. For example, with a range of $28 to $40 for group therapy for master's-level clinicians who are paid $48 to $75 for individual therapy, the pay is better with six patients at $28 in a group session than with one individual at $48 per hour (Tuttle, 1995).

Q How can I sell group therapy? Where does the money come from for the marketing?

A Start with a simple table listing therapy groups, the clinicians who lead the groups, specialty areas, times and locations offered, and prices. The difficult thing about offering a menu of therapy groups is that you have to sustain a certain amount of volume. The best marketing tool in this case is a flier. Use a standard format with different colors for different groups. Desktop publishing layout costs about $15 per hour, and it should take no more than one hour per flier. Reproduced in batches of 50 or 100 at a budget printer, the fliers are attached to letters mailed to managed care firms.

Group therapy fliers are good eye-catchers among case managers, who often come from community mental health backgrounds. Having an attractive menu of therapy groups is a good selling point with managed care firms moving to case rates—and a must for providers to be able to balance costs under the new pricing plans. (See Exhibit 5.4.)

MARKETING PLANS

Q As I prepare for managed care, are there particular areas of my practice that I should consider?

A Try this checklist offered by Tracy Todd of the Brief Therapy Institute of Denver as a guide to your practice assessment (Todd, 1994):

- Define quality: Are you meeting your customers' needs—both clients and payers?
- Make service flexible to meet market demands.

EXHIBIT 5.4. Marketing Plans for Therapy Groups.

1. Describe on a single page each therapy group offered by the practice, including treatment goals.
2. List possible clients for each group.
3. Cluster the therapy groups around several diagnosis or problem categories, such as chemically dependent patients, adolescent substance abuse, parent group for substance abuse, attention deficit/hyperactivity disorder (ADHD), latency age group, parents' group, adolescent group, and adult group.
4. Poll third-party payer case managers and community referral sources to find needs that match your offering, or ideas for new groups. Examples are:
   - School counselors—attention deficit disorder socialization groups
   - Clergy—bereavement
   - Primary care doctors — pain management
   - Ob-gyns — new parent groups
5. Use the contacts to offer public speaking or introductory sessions.

Source: Developed by Mark Dworkin, LCSW, BCD, Long Island, NY.

- Aim to decrease costs, while increasing your menu of services and access (hours, locations).
- Streamline administration; look hard at office management.
- How fast can you respond to the market? Are applications and credentials in order?
- How quickly can you see new patients?

Q I'm on several managed care panels, but I see very few referrals. How do I get more patients?

A Large specialty managed care firms maintain panels of between 20,000 and 35,000 providers, but nearly 80% of referrals are going to about 25% of the panel providers. Those panels are expected to shrink by about 20%, and more referrals will be going to large, structured group practices. Some referrals are based on which providers the case managers know. Other firms make referrals on the basis of complicated profiling systems that rank providers by utilization, length of treatment, cost of services, patient satisfaction, case management satisfaction, and red flags warning of critical incidents or repeat hospital admissions.

Here are some steps that providers can take to increase their chances of attracting case manager referrals.

1. Target two or three of the managed care firms with employer-clients in your area. Then ask the case managers of those firms to look at your provider profile. Tell the case managers that you would like to receive more referrals and that you're seeking information to help make you more attractive. Your profile may list too many specialities, or not enough. If you're listed as a generalist, ask the case manager about the company's specialist needs. Popular requests are for providers who work with children, those with attention deficit hyperactivity disorder (ADHD), hearing-impaired patients, and different ethnic and religious populations.
2. Once you're sure that your profile lists correct information that meets the managed care firm's needs, consider using a quarterly newsletter to keep case managers and EAPs informed about new services. Some groups send a simple update to their top five managed care firms showing new hours, therapy groups, group meeting times, or psychoeducational workshops. Newsletters work best with smaller

regional managed care firms or EAPs, or when case managers already know the provider.

3. Learn which large group practices in your community have "preferred provider" arrangements with managed care firms. Those groups are receiving the majority of referrals and use other individual providers as part of their own networks. Go directly to the large groups and ask what specialties they lack and how you can be a part of their referral chain.
4. Use your patient satisfaction survey results as a sales tool. One group practice used charts and graphs to illustrate patient approval as part of its marketing materials. Another practice keeps its finger on managed care's pulse with a customer satisfaction survey that's also sent to referring primary care physicians and EAPs. See examples in Appendix E.

Q Will adding evening and weekend hours increase my referrals?

A There's a good chance that it will, that is, if you let the managed care firm know about your new hours. Better yet, talk to the case manager first and ask: Are there hours when it is difficult for your client's employees to find a therapist? Then offer to add those hours to your schedule—perhaps Saturday mornings, Sunday afternoons, before-work hours, or after-work hours. The idea is to make it easier for clients to keep appointments without missing any more work than is absolutely necessary.

Q Should I pay to get on a managed care panel?

A Some regional provider-managed care networks charge a low fee ($50 to $200) to cover credentialing and to offset some administrative overhead. It can be a wise investment, especially if it is a way to diversify your market efforts to include direct employer contracting.

Be very wary, however, of direct mail promises of contracts and referrals in exchange for dollars. Chances are, they're building a provider list for use in marketing to employers. Ask whether the network has actual contracts with employers or other payers. Ask for names, addresses, and telephone numbers. Request a provider list. Contact other providers in your community and ask if they have received referrals.

Q I don't have time to go to business association meetings. How can I make the contacts?

A This may be a case of needing to make the time to do something important for your practice. If you can commit to one business networking event each week, that's a start. One group practice sets aside each Monday at noon to invite representatives from a hospital, facility, primary care physician's office, managed care company and/or EAP for box lunches. It only takes an hour and the idea is to learn more about the visitors, not to promote the practice. That comes later.

Another possibility is to join a statewide Chamber of Commerce or business organization and offer to serve on the health insurance committee. Or offer a representative from your professional association. Local chambers usually have monthly "after hours," or social events. That's a good time to listen to employer concerns in an informal setting and to schedule lunch appointments during the month to talk more about how you might help address those concerns.

Exhibit 5.5 lists 10 market leads and Exhibit 5.6 identifies 15 steps that you can take to establish yourself in new markets.

Q When completing a managed care panel application, should I check as many specialties as possible?

A No. Look at the checklist and think first of those areas in which you really are exceptionally skilled, those that set you apart from other community providers. Then think in terms of those skills that are covered by benefit packages. This isn't the time to lobby for inclusion of your pet therapy under coverage. Rather, indicate two or three strong specialties in which you are proficient, the services are covered, and that you are pretty certain they are not already offered by your competitors.

Q What if the panel is closed?

A There's no such thing as a closed panel. Managed care provider networks are amorphous. They shrink and expand as the companies

EXHIBIT 5.5. Critical Market Research for Managed Care: 10 Market Leads to Track Tomorrow.

1. **State insurance commissioners and regulatory boards.**
   Know the 10 largest managed care firms doing business in your state. Know which companies are regulated and for what services.
2. **State business alliances or chambers of commerce.**
   Buy their membership directories. Know the 10 largest employers in your area. Find out what benefits they offer, where they buy the services, and what they need.
3. **Local chambers of commerce.**
   Know the middle-sized and small employers and whether they are part of purchasing alliances.
4. **State and local health planning organizations.**
   Professional associations usually have representatives and can tell you when they meet.
5. **Employee Assistance Program providers.**
   Nationally, EAPA can provide a listing. Contact state chapters to buy local lists.
6. **Business journals and trade associations.**
   These groups sell mailing lists on labels or disks. Most break them out by location, size of company, and number of employees, and some include insurance coverage data.
7. **Yellow Pages.**
   Who is already selling what you want to offer? Know the competition. Know potential alliances.
8. **Local contract agencies.**
   Call on school systems, courts, county and city governments. Look for areas where budget cuts have created openings for contract work. Ask about needs, and then be creative with new services. Look for ways to generate referrals as an alternative to sentencing, school suspensions, or employer disciplinary actions.
9. **Industry publications.**
   Watch for requests for proposal (RFPs) and new contracts. Know national contracts and their local clients and be ahead of the pack.
10. **Industrial development commissions.**
    Talk to recruiters. Know about new companies before they arrive.

Source: Market Leads. Gayle Tuttle & Associates, Inc., Clayton, NC.

EXHIBIT 5.6. Developing Products for New Markets: 15 Steps You Can Take Tomorrow.

1. **Build name recognition.**

   Don't assume that referral sources know about you or what you do. Providers are going back to tried-and-true public speaking and freebie workshops to establish themselves in even heavy managed care communities. Having a client ask for you by name can open an otherwise closed network panel.

2. **Set yourself apart.**

   Take a hard look at your clinical specialties. Review you background and define what you do well. Consider adding one thing to your practice that no one else in your geographic area is offering.

3. **Set up alternative levels of care.**

   Be creative. Ask chemical dependency facilities what outpatient services they need. What about mobile outreach or evening programs? Can you use the facility for a partial program?

4. **Know the players.**

   Who are the managed care companies doing business in your area? With which employers do they contract? Which employers are self-insured and are willing to contract directly with provider groups?

5. **Practice business skills.**

   Do you know how to measure the cost of your services?

6. **Use outcomes data.**

   Measure your client/patient satisfaction. Show buyers that you are willing to measure your services, and that your practice has proven results.

7. **Take a hard look at your marketing materials.**

   Do they highlight specialty services that an employer or managed care firm might buy separately? Consider a marketing package that can be easily tailored to various clients. Use inserts that can be changed inexpensively to target employers, managed care, traditional referral sources, primary care physicians, and private-pay clients.

8. **Know your community resources.**

   Be willing to offer competent group therapy and to step down to community support programs.

9. **Put someone in charge of managed care business.**

   Train a case manager within the practice to handle relationships with managed care firms and to provide immediate feedback on patients in treatment.

10. **Join a Chamber of Commerce.**

    Volunteer to serve on an insurance or health care committee as a way to win a seat at the benefits table. Offer your services as a resource for employers in designing programs to comply with the Drug Free Workplace Act, Workers' Compensation guidelines, and the Americans with Disabilities Act.

11. **Set aside one day each week to order box lunches and invite a managed care firm, local hospital, psychiatric facility, or employer to visit your practice. Pay close attention to learn their functions and their needs.**

12. **Rethink your program's pricing strategies.**

    Select two or three services as "products" and attach competitive case rate or other package prices.

13. **Ask a friend who works for a major employer to help set up a "focus" group with interested employees to provide feedback on one of your products.**

    Provide box lunches. Ask the group these questions: Do you need this product? How much would you pay? How many sessions would you commit to? Would you be interested in the service if it were offered at the work site?

14. **Think Access.**

    Take the show on the road and be willing to provide care in affordable blocks of sessions in schools, in doctor's offices, and at work sites.

15. **Talk to other professionals about their needs.**

    Cross-refer with your lawyer, doctor, or investment broker. Be willing to identify client needs for other professional services and make referrals.

Source: Marketing Checklist. Gayle Tuttle & Associates, Clayton, NC.

win and lose employer contracts. Never write off a firm. While it may not need new providers today, chances are that it will tomorrow.

Consider a slightly different question when approaching a provider relations director: Do you have special network needs? Nearly every managed care firm needs child psychiatrists. And rarely will one turn away bicultural, bilingual providers, or those who can communicate through sign language. That may not establish you as a "bull's-eye" provider where you can count on the firm for 80% of your business, but it will get you in the door and allow you to build a relationship.

If the company doesn't currently need providers, leave the door open. Set up a tickle file, and look for reasons to be in touch a few weeks or months later. Watch the newspaper for new industries coming to town. Learn about their workers and needs. Approach the managed care firm as a partner in attracting new businesses. Remember that the people working for managed care firms appreciate clinicians who are interested in helping them do a better job.

Q How much should I spend on marketing?

A In terms of time, the number most often mentioned is 20%. For a single provider, that's one full day each week, based on a 40-hour week. There is no industry standard for market dollars.

Q Is it too late? Are there any openings? I feel as though I need to know more than I can learn.

A The answer is location, location, location. It may be too late in some areas. California is a good example, where 60,000 of the nation's 360,000 licensed therapists are practicing. Other saturated areas are New York and Chicago and the states of Florida and Arizona. Major metropolitan areas are especially tight, whereas managed care firms are recruiting providers for rural areas.

While panels are sometimes filled to meet existing contracts, managed care needs change as the companies gain and lose employer clients. Although tracking the industry can seem overwhelming, providers have the best shot at managing their practices when they narrow their focus to the local market. Keeping the list short can make it more manageable.

- Who are the 10 largest employers in your area?
- Which managed care firm holds the contract for their behavioral health coverage?
- What is the makeup of the employee population?
- What special needs might they have?
- What skills do you have that might meet those needs?
- What does the managed care firm need to enhance its services to the employer?
- What new industries are coming to your area?

Q What about satellite offices? I've been told that managed care firms will add providers if they open offices in outlying communities. Is this true?

A It all depends on the managed care firm's need to service its employer clients in your area. Before opening an additional office, providers should research the local market. Talk to case managers at managed care firms to learn about new contracts with outlying employers. Ask them if clients from certain areas have to drive more than 20 miles to reach a provider. Is there enough volume to make it worth your while? What about sharing a satellite office with another provider, say, a physical therapist or occupational therapist, and offering part-time hours? Is the managed care firm willing to guarantee a set number of referrals to help support your expansion? Are there other providers already offering the same services in those areas? Are there services you offer that those providers need, and would they be willing to share part-time space in order to increase referrals?

Q What kind of marketing materials do I need?

A Concentrate on simple brochures that tell managed care firms who you are, where you are located, the types of services you offer, and your office hours. Most provider relations directors aren't interested in expensive, glossy packages that include listings of professional papers. Many providers hire a graphics designer to help them put together a neat, well-written brochure that can be produced on inexpensive preprinted papers (that is, papers with preprinted color and design for personal computer use). This allows printing of only as many as are needed. Have the brochure designed on universal software and keep a copy on diskette along with a camera-ready version that can be reproduced at a budget printer.

Consider a pocket brochure with inserts that can be added or removed for special markets, including employers, EAPs, primary care physicians, and HMOs.

Q How can I get referrals from a group that already has preferred managed care status? Is that a better idea than starting on my own?

A For solo and very small group practices, marketing to larger group practices is a very good strategy for increasing managed care market share. Get to know the high-volume groups—those with preferred relationships with managed care firms—in your area. They are challenged to offer as broad a continuum of services as possible. Often adding your specialty services, flexible hours, and programs to their package enhances a group's position and makes a lot more economic sense than developing its own. Those groups are doing very much the same thing that managed care firms did when they first developed provider panels. Strengthening referral relationships with colleagues who may have been viewed as competitors in an earlier market can balance a practice mix for a small group and allow its members to concentrate on private pay and direct contract marketing.

Q What provider qualities do managed care firms view as enhancing?

A They look for patience, respect for case managers and the role of the managed care firm, the ability to communicate clearly with case managers, willingness to use computers and technology to ease the paperwork burden, and the willingness and ability to write clear and concise treatment reports.

Managed care firms aren't put off by a provider who is assertive on behalf of patients as long as the request is handled politely, and as long as the provider understands the limits of the employee's benefit plan. Most case managers appreciate providers who return their calls quickly, or set aside a time each day when they can be reached to discuss treatment plans. A last note is that case managers are impressed with providers who know and are willing to refer to community resources when appropriate. Marjorie Nichols, a provider who has worked inside managed care firms and now consults with both MCOs and providers, lists three qualities that are critical in impressing case managers: speaking the same language when discussing treatment plans, being easy to access and available to accept referrals, and responding promptly to case manager calls (Nichols, 1994).

Q I'm on several managed care panels, but I see very few referrals. How do I get more patients?

A Managed care firms responding to national surveys report an average of 10 new referrals per provider per year, but providers responding to surveys report an average of three new referrals from each managed care contract. Merit Behavioral Care Corporation has said that 70% of its referrals go to 25% of its national network of more than 20,000 providers. So, the low number of new referrals is in line.

Where are the referrals going? They're going to multidisciplinary group practices that have achieved partnerships with managed care firms as key, anchor, or preferred providers. They adhere to the companies' treatment guidelines, act as gatekeepers providing assessment and referral services themselves, and get first crack at patients not treated in staff model clinics. For credentialed providers on the outer rim of managed care's bull's-eye, the marketing target becomes the larger group practice in your area. Approach groups as a resource that will allow them to expand their one-stop shopping through your specialties. (See Exhibit 5.7.)

EXHIBIT 5.7. Managed Care Triggers for Referrals.

Specialties
Age
Sex
Minority representation
Distance/drive time
Community reputation
Group practices
Bicultural/bilingual capability

Q How do I know what my competitors are doing?

A First, don't assume that other clinicians, group practices, partial programs, day treatment programs, or facilities are competitors. Yesterday's competitor could very well be your friend in today's integrated market. As you acquire information about other providers, sift and sort it for relationship potential as well as competition.

Newspapers: Look at classified job listings to learn about expansions and new products, as well as display ads promoting programs to employers. Check the free calendar listings of local shoppers for open-house opportunities at new facilities, programs, and group practices.

Open houses: Go or send a staffer to open-house opportunities at other provider groups, programs, and facilities. Bring back brochures, therapy group schedules, and directories of clinicians with specialty skills.

Managed care contacts: Network with your referral sources to learn what's new in the market. They'll know about mergers, acquisitions, and newcomers. Share tidbits regularly to keep the information coming.

Yellow Pages ads: Browse the Yellow Pages to see what other programs are listed as services.

Clients: Listen to your clients. What programs did they hear about or consider before coming to you? Check your marketing by asking at intake how they learned about your practice. The most important marketing research that a provider can do takes place in his or her own office. Go to your files and look at your referral sources and patterns. Where is your business coming from? What do you know about the companies that employ most of your clients?

Q How can I work with primary care doctors?

A A major industry trend is the return of behavioral health care to HMOs. Disease management templates have been developed for asthma, HIV, cardiac rehabilitation, cancer, and chronic pain include psychotherapy. Regional HMOs are recruiting therapists to place in the offices of their primary group practices for medication consultations and immediate referrals.

Behavioral group practices are linking with primary care practices as part of integrated delivery systems. (See Exhibit 5.8.)

A growing number of providers are locating their practices in the offices of gynecologists, pediatricians, and family practitioners. Others are in clinics with physical and occupational therapists, or work with plastic surgeons and dentists. One therapist specializing in hypnosis works with a urologist. The key to successful relationships with doctors, they agree, is to break out of the 50-minute-session mold. (See Exhibit 5.9.)

Providers working with primary care doctors say that they see more patients during 15-minute examining room consultations and have a number of referrals for one or two sessions.

EXHIBIT 5.8. Recommended Consults.

Frequent office visits or phone calls
Prescription of psychotropic medications
Diagnosis of alcohol or other drug abuse
Diagnosis of eating disorder
Reported sexual problems
Diagnosis of sexually transmitted disease
Diagnosis of pregnancy or request for abortion
Reported couples' problems
Reported family violence
Victims of rape and their family members
Questions about school discipline
Termination of care
Recommendation of nursing home placement
Request for counseling referral
Diagnosis of any chronic illness
Chronic abdominal pain
Chronic pelvic pain
Chronic fatigue
Headaches
Insomnia
School problems, including suspected ADHD
Adolescents with family or other problems
Death of a family member
Diagnosis of anxiety or panic disorder
Diagnosis of depression
Chronic noncompliance
Consideration of obesity
Smoking

Source: Anthony Heath. MacNeal Family Practice Residency. Berwyn, IL. Reprinted with permission.

EXHIBIT 5.9. How to Work with Medical Doctors.

Location, location, location
Be easily accessible by phone
Carry a pager during office hours
Always be brief and succinct
Provide ongoing and prompt feedback
Offer to document visits in patients' charts
Use SOAP format for charting
Do and provide genograms for all patients
Demonstrate knowledge of DSM-IV
Demonstrate knowledge of psychotropic medications
Refer patients to physicians for physicals and medications

Source: Anthony Heath. MacNeal Family Practice Residency. Berwyn, IL. Reprinted with permission.

REFERENCES

Martin, K., & Tuttle, G. M. (1994, June). Do's and don'ts of working with a consultant. Presented at *Psychotherapy Finances'* second annual Managed Care Conference.

Nichols, M. (1994, May). Nuts and bolts: Working effectively with managed care. Presented at a meeting of the North Carolina Society for Clinical Social Work.

Todd, T. (1994). Fitting market trends to your practice. Presented at a meeting of the American Association for Marriage and Family Therapy.

Tuttle, G. (1995). Practice looks to group therapy to cut clinical hours, boost pay. *Practice Strategies, 1*(2).

Tuttle, G. (1996). Making cure rates work. *Practice Strategies, 2*(1), 1.

6

Life After Managed Care

> The fact is, there is no little black box; it's all a marketing gimmick. Everyone is doing the same thing, only now everyone knows how to do it—including the providers.
>
> *Nicholas A. Cummings, Ph.D., Sc.D.*

Nicholas A. Cummings, a controversial past president of the American Psychological Association, has drawn criticism, envy, and always an audience since he first predicted that managed care would permeate mental health and substance abuse treatment.

Again in the role of a soothsayer, Cummings was ahead of the curve when he began forecasting the demise of the behavioral health carve-out industry that he helped to create by founding American Biodyne, now part of the Merit Behavioral Care Corporation. "Carve-outs are over," he has said flatly, with a clear warning that therapists should act quickly to compete directly with the beleaguered specialty companies. "You can compete because they are hurting badly" (Tuttle, 1996d).

Many large group practices that followed the recipes for success as shared by managed care carve-out firms are agreeing with Cummings. Owners of premier practices who were counting on partnerships with managed care firms to keep their businesses strong say the protection they hoped for was illusionary. "We're being penalized for our successes," says Neil Dickman, Ph.D., the CEO of Pacific Applied Psychology Associates in Berkeley, Calif. (Tuttle, 1996c). Large practice owners are spending hundreds of thousands of dollars each year on quality assurance programs, state-of-the-art computer tracking systems, and large support staffs to perform administrative tasks that once were the chores of managed care firms, and reporting monthly financial losses while clinicians are seeing more patients. "This has become an industry that's eating its young," says Jeffrey Simon, Ph.D., the president of Carmel Psychological Associates, PC, in Carmel, N.Y. "I defy any other business to take these losses and keep going" (private interview).

Practicing in a new era of consumer awareness, measured results, and increased accountability, clinicians realize they can't return to old methods. The result is a sophisticated pool of therapists with refined clinical skills who are looking for creative ways to reduce their dependence on carve-out firms. Some are vehemently opposed to all forms of managed care, while other clinicians are mimicking the shape and form of the industry in provider-driven networks.

Coauthor Dianne Rush Woods offers this example of a provider's response to price squeezes and administrative burdens:

> As a director of provider relations, I once received a resignation letter from a therapist who stated:
>
> > I'm resigning from your network because I find working with managed care too cumbersome. The fees are too small and the paperwork incredibly onerous. But, I am not quitting without a plan. Here's the plan.
> >
> > I am reducing my fees to $50 per hour, which is about what I make after I deduct all the time spent on paperwork and phone calls with managed care. I will advertise my reduced rates and increase my volume of lower-paying patients.
> >
> > I will market to local businesses and schools for clients who will be able to afford to pay these lower fees. I can then do what I've been trained to do, rather than being retrained by you.

The key for this clinician was a willingness to make the necessary changes in her practice and pricing in order to be competitive. There's no shortage of providers who want to escape managed care for a private-pay market. But many clinicians are unwilling to see that rising HMO enrollment and competition among managed care firms have driven prices down. "A lot of people are doing things out of fear, but not because they have made a decision to proactively take care of their practice," says Michael Bowers, M.A., executive director of the American Association for Marriage and Family Therapy (Karuth, 1996).

Clinicians who attract a new private-pay clientele are adjusting the rates down to the $40 to $60 range. They're negotiating case rates and expanding their views of therapeutic intervention to include psychoeducational groups, multifamily groups, couples retreats, school consultations, support groups for chronically ill patients, and working with health care providers.

PRACTICE DIVERSIFICATION

Q Is there a private-pay market for individual practitioners?

A Alan Savitz, M.D., the CEO of PacifiCare Behavioral Health, has joked that the private-pay market will be similar to cosmetic surgery. "That might not be too bad," he says. "All the plastic surgeons seem to be doing well and driving big cars" (Savitz, 1993).

Yes, there will be a private-pay market. The strength of that market will vary with its location and the ability to pay in any given setting. Predictions for the private-pay market range from 2% to 15%. Psychologists are banking on individuals to shop for higher credentials and licensing when paying out-of-pocket for services not covered by third-party payers. Other providers are looking for ways to package services to make them affordable, such as flat rates for a set number of couples therapy sessions.

An increasing number of therapists are banding together to offer their services outside of managed care, and most of these groups are lowering their fees to become competitive with managed care.

Q How are those groups different from managed care?

A In many cases, provider-sponsored delivery systems are very much like managed care firms. The goal for most is to eliminate the third-party carve-out firm, and contract directly with employers, hospitals, physician groups, HMOs and insurers to manage and deliver behavioral health care. They are trying to capture the dollar that is now paid to managed behavioral health care firms.

Q How much are carve-out firms paid?

A Large group practices tell us they are receiving an average of 25 to 30% of the dollar paid by employers for mental health and substance abuse services. The balance remains with the carve-out firms. There's growing frustration on the part of large group practices that have taken on expensive administrative responsibilities and find themselves receiving fees comparable to those paid to solo practitioners.

Q Is there a guarantee that providers can recover that difference if they bypass carve-out firms?

A Not at all. In fact, one group practice delivering services to an HMO through a carve-out firm recently negotiated to provide the same services directly to the HMO. The HMO offered a rate 18% lower than the group was receiving under its existing carve-out contract.

Q What is the point of marketing to HMOs and payers if the fees will continue to drop?

A The key is for the practice to achieve a diversified payer mix. Management of care is inevitable and employers who are going to include behavioral care as part of their benefits are going to demand that costs and services be monitored. Providers who are able to contract directly with the employer, or with the patient for private pay, will have more control over pricing. Local economies and competitive market forces, however, will determine price. HMOs reported an increase in membership of 7.7 million last year, for a total enrollment of nearly 54 million (Interstudy, Minneapolis, Minn.). Providers who want a share of the business held by managed care firms, including HMOs, may have few choices in pricing for those customers.

A New York provider, for example, balked at lower rates when Prudential contracted with Value Behavioral Health and Merit Behavioral Care Corporation to assume its behavioral health services under capitated contracts. A representative of one of the carve-outs cautioned the provider to consider, before giving up her panel slot, that she could expect similar price drops under contracts with other HMOs. Dropping out now, the company representative warned, could block her from receiving additional referrals.

Q So, it's take it or leave it?

A In some cases, yes. Generally, the answer is not that cut and dried. Again, local market factors and provider awareness of the cost of doing business must be considered in each case. If the company has a greater need for a certain specialty or provider discipline in a geographic area, the provider will have more bargaining power. Keep in mind that 25,000 people will complete graduate programs in mental health fields in 1997 (Marques, 1993). They will join more than 300,000 licensed clinicians. It's exactly this sort of ultimatum, however, that is impelling providers to form their own delivery systems and attempt to compete for local employer and private patient business.

Q What about fighting back through lawsuits and legislation?

A State associations of providers have focused much of their energy on any-willing-provider (AWP) legislation. More than 20 states have passed some form of AWP laws that address behavioral health providers and require managed care firms to include on panels those clinicians meeting their requirements and willing to accept their fees. Getting on panels, however, has little to do with receiving referrals.

The emphasis has shifted now to state legislation to regulate how managed care firms do business, and to set guidelines for notifying providers of panel decisions. A number of lawyers are gathering examples of provider discrimination and complaints for possible class action lawsuits.

But those methods address the future, and many providers are worried that they may not still be in business when and if legislative and legal remedies are instituted. A leader in the fight against managed behavioral care has been Karen Shore through her National Coalition of Mental Health Professionals and Consumers, Inc. (Karuth, 1996). Based in New York, the coalition has 17 affiliated state organizations and a few dozen affiliated groups nationwide. Its purpose is to expose abuses under managed care, and to support legislation to regulate the industry and to eliminate employer-paid coverage, returning the money to consumers through tax-free bank accounts. "We need a system that allows consumer freedom," says Shore. "The only way is if they take responsibility for their costs" (private interview).

Shore's approach is one of absolute opposition to managed care as an industry. Providers who don't like working for managed care are divided between those who openly shun the carve-out firms and those who want the best of both markets. The coalition can be reached by writing to Shore at P.O. Box 438, Commack, NY 11725-0438.

Q Are there examples of providers who are resisting managed care in their practices?

A One example is the Manassas Group in Roanoke, Va., led by psychologist Dana Ackley. "My personal view," Ackley says, "is that if managed care wants the business, they can have it. I prefer to do therapy. My view of the future is to move outside of third-party reimbursement. I am not on any managed care panels. I never intend to be" (private interview).

The Manassas Group is structured as a group-without-walls, similar to early practices created to sell services to managed care firms. Individual practitioners pay a fee to a corporation owned by Ackley and two other group members for office space, a receptionist, and billing services. Some of the therapists are providers for managed care firms, or work for hospitals that contract with managed care companies—but not through referrals from the Manassas Group. Ackley relies on traditional market research to sell consulting and clinical services directly to employers, as well as to private pay clients. He leads workshops on "Building a Managed Care Free Practice" that show clinicians how to use the best of what carve-out firms can teach them to run independent practices. That includes offering financing options to make it easier for individuals to afford his services. He continues to charge $95 for 50-minute sessions.

Q Are there examples of financing options?

A Some such examples are discounts for clients who don't use their insurance coverage and for those who pay in full at each session; lines of credit of up to $1,000, with a partial payment up front and interest charges; set rates for a number of sessions, with discounts for payment in advance, or higher rates when divided into two or three payments; and acceptance of general-use credit cards.

Q How can providers sell directly to individuals without jeopardizing managed care contracts?

A Providers should read their managed care contracts carefully to determine whether they have agreed not to offer out-of-pocket options to managed care clients. Feeling the crunch of managed care fee reductions and the increased overhead, many clinicians are much less worried about how managed care firms may react than about going out of business.

Ginger Blume, a Connecticut psychologist who holds a number of managed care contracts, offers referrals the option of private-pay appointments when she does not have a provider credentialed and available under the client's plan. So far, there's been no managed care backlash.

"I tell them that if they can't find another therapist under their plan who is available at the time they need, give us a call back and we'll see you out-of-pocket" (Tuttle, 1996a). She uses a brochure stressing the option, and reminding clients of managed care negatives, including the release of confidential information to claims reviewers and case managers. She is strict about patient payments, insisting that money be received at the beginning of each session. Clients who forget their checkbooks must pay at the beginning of the next session or therapy is not continued.

Q Are providers of several disciplines working together to offer alternatives to managed care?

A Yes. A variety of systems involve providers working outside of managed care. Some have been more successful than others, and some are still in their infancy. One of the earliest attempts to market collectively outside managed care was the Boulder Psychotherapists Guild in Colorado, which in 1993 started offering private-pay clients a 20% discount (Tuttle, 1994). Another, known as the San Fernando Valley Alliance of Mental Health Professionals for the Preservation of Privacy and Self-Determination in Psychotherapy, offered lower fees and sliding scales in an effort to draw patients away from managed care firms (Karuth, 1996). The marketing efforts were unsuccessful and some alliance members are now eyeing a therapist-owned capitated system.

The American Mental Health Alliance in Massachusetts charges $400 to $600 to help providers in other states develop cooperatives for bidding on government and business contracts (Bailey, 1996). Some members of the alliance refuse to work with managed care, while others are network providers. Providers are paid on a sliding scale, with full fees for the first two sessions and lower payments for additional sessions. They are responsible for collecting co-payments.

Groups of marriage and family therapists in Oregon, Massachusetts, and Tennessee are developing statewide systems outside their professional associations for credentialing networks of providers to market to employers. Another example is the Pennsylvania Community Providers Association. In Huntington, N.Y., nearly 200 psychologists have paid $4,000 each to join a provider-owned HMO of 2,000 physicians (Saeman, 1996).

Q What is the difference for providers contracting as individuals with provider-owned systems and with managed care systems?

A Most provider-owned delivery systems have evolved from large group practices. Keep in mind that as those groups are questioning the value of their partnerships with managed care firms, they are hearing the same questions from individuals in networks designed to help handle referrals. They are working harder for less. On the whole, however, providers contracting with clinician-owned systems can expect more referrals in a year, and somewhat higher fees (Tuttle, 1996b). In responses by eight such systems to a national industry survey, the groups reported 15% more referrals to providers than are made by carve-out firms. Provider-owned systems tend to include more master's-level therapists and fees tend to flatten across discipline lines rather than favoring M.D.'s and psychologists.

Q Are there services that I should add to my practice in order to attract private-pay clients?

A The answer depends on the customers in your particular market. In addition to reducing fees for traditional therapy in order to attract patients who choose not to access benefits, many therapists are banking on services that aren't covered by insurance or managed care plans. For example, a Florida practice offers wellness products by adding massage therapists, nutritionists, and hypnotherapists to its clinical staff. Executive coaching and business consulting services for employers are other options. Weight control, stress management, relaxation techniques, communication skills, and support groups for new mothers all are examples of fixed-price, time-limited services being offered to out-of-pocket clients.

REFERENCES

Bailey, L. (1996). Provider co-ops hope to bypass managed care. *Practice Strategies, 2*(6), 7–8.

Karuth, L. (1996, May/June). Providers confront the future: How are therapists responding to managed care? *Behavioral Health Management*, pp. 10–13.

Marques, C. (1993). Are we training too many mental health providers? *Behavioral Healthcare Tomorrow, 2*(6), 26–28.

Saeman, H. (1996). 280 Long Island psychologists join 2,000 physicians in provider-owned HMO. *National Psychologist, 5*(1), 6.

Savitz, A. (1993, June). Future Trends. Presentation to Psychotherapy Finances Managed Care Conference.

Tuttle, G. (1994). Marketing: Cutting prices to attract self-pay clients. *Psychotherapy Finances, 20*(2), 1–2.

Tuttle, G. (1996a). Catch-22: Too little, too late; too much, too soon. *Practice Strategies, 2*(7), 1– 9.

Tuttle, G., (1996b). Colleagues pay higher fees, make more referrals. *Practice Strategies, 2*(8), 6–7.

Tuttle, G. (1996c). Premier group practices cry foul on managed care squeeze. *Practice Strategies, 2*(9), 1, 2, 9.

Tuttle, G. (1996d). Will Merit exit slam the lid on managed care's black box? *Practice Strategies, 2*(2), 1–2.

APPENDIX A

GLOSSARY

Anchor Group (also known as core groups, preferred groups, clinical regional groups): Large multidisciplinary provider groups offering a broad menu of services to provide one-stop shopping for managed care firms. The group might consist of one or more psychiatrists, several psychologists, a clinical social worker, marriage and family counselors, and a clinical nurse specialist. The group typically has special relationships with managed care companies that accept lower fees for increased referrals. There may be an exclusive or semiexclusive relationship with one or more managed care companies. Managed care firms have groomed the groups to provide utilization review, case management, quality assurance, intake and referral, and outcomes measurement and reporting services, thus allowing the companies to reduce operating costs.

Any Willing Provider Law: Laws that allow states to require the inclusion of any willing provider who is qualified and meets the credentialing standards of the managed care organization. These laws have been vigorously supported by state and national professional organizations, which their members shut out by managed care organizations with "closed panels".

At Risk: A term used to describe a financial arrangement in health care financing. In traditional indemnity plans, the insurance company was at risk for any claims that exceeded the premium revenue. In managed care arrangements, risk is increasingly assumed by providers. Risk can be shared, or, in the case of fully capitated contracts, the provider may be at full risk. State insurance licensing laws determine the extent to which provider groups may assume risk.

Capitation: A prepaid plan based on a set number of covered lives under a defined benefits package. Payments are made to the provider in monthly advances, rather than as fees for services provided.

Capitation Rate: The amount of monthly reimbursement per covered life in a capitated contract, often referred to as the "pmpm" (or per member, per month) reimbursement rate. This model specifies a dollar amount negotiated by the payer and the provider to cover the cost of services for a group of people.

Carve-In: The return of specialized behavioral health care services to HMOs and general health insurance plans.

Carve-Out: Separating the management and delivery of a set of health care services from general health care benefits. In behavioral health care, this means the assignment of mental health and chemical dependency utilization review and management to companies specializing in those areas. A mental health "carve-out" company specializes in providing mental health services to individuals whose medical services are covered under other plans.

Case Management: The overseeing of treatment delivery through the continuum of care. This process involves concurrent and retrospective review.

Case Rate: A plan offering one payment regardless of the number of episodes of treatment. The provider receives a set rate whether it provides one session of care or 20. The decision about the number of sessions is left to the provider, who decides what amount of clinical care is needed to treat the presenting problem under a benefits plan.

Coinsurance: The amount of payment for which the covered enrollee is responsible. Typically, the plan pays 80% for the insurance benefit and the covered enrollee or beneficiary pays 20%. Therefore, if your contract rate is $80 and the coinsurance rate is 20%, excluding deductibles (which are defined below), the insurance company pays $60 and the enrollee or beneficiary pays $20.

Continuum of Care: A program that ensures that uninterrupted care is available and provided at the appropriate level of intensity—from inpatient, to partial, to intensive or once-a-week outpatient treatment. This continuum is being offered more frequently by partnerships between hospital systems and behavioral health care systems, as well as partnerships between large primary care physician groups and behavioral health care IPAs, Groups Without Walls, or consortiums of group practices.

Copayment: That portion of a claims payment for which the covered enrollee or beneficiary is responsible. This is the flat rate amount a member must pay upon receiving covered health care services. In some instances, the covered enrollee has a $0 copayment for the first five sessions; sessions 6–10 have a $10 copayment, sessions 11–20 have a $20 copayment, and sessions 21+ have a copayment of $30.

Cost Offset: Savings achieved in medical benefits dollars through the treatment of mental illness, chemical dependency, or behavioral disorders. For example, these include savings achieved in the treatment of cardiac and major illness as a result of behavioral therapy as a part of weight control, or savings in medical treatment of chronic pain through biofeedback.

Covered Enrollee or Covered Life: An individual who is covered under a benefit plan. However, a person may be employed and not be an eligible, covered life. Or the employee may be eligible but his or her spouse or children may not be considered covered lives.

Deductible: The amount of money that must be paid, out-of-pocket, by the covered enrollee before the benefit is activated. Recently, there has been a steep increase in deductibles, specifically in reference to inpatient hospitalization, which effectively diminishes access for a number of covered enrollees (they cannot afford the initial out-of-pocket cost). Therefore, a person may have a $200 deductible (this is often for all medical benefits, including medical, mental health, and chemical dependency) that must be met before that person is covered by his or her benefit. It is important for clinicians to differentiate clearly between copayment, coinsurance, and deductible by seeking preauthorization and benefits clarification prior to providing care.

Employee Assistance Program (EAP): A program established to provide clinical services that attempt to identify and solve work performance and common life problems. It may offer assessment, referral, follow-up, chemical dependency assessment, and brief counseling. Such plans can be managed internally within the corporation, by external EAP speciality companies or by managed care corporations. Increasingly, EAPs provide a limited number of brief therapy sessions. Other add-ons offered through some EAPs include legal, financial, and child-care referral services.

Point of Service (POS): An open-ended plan that allows for choice in the selection of benefits. Copayments are lower under tight benefit management. The greater the choice, the higher is the cost of copayment for the covered enrollee.

Preferred Provider Organization (PPO): Companies that organize their own network of providers to deliver services and establish fees; an organization of independent providers joined to offer discounted, fee-for-service managed care contracting. It is usually a separate entity, owned by some or all of the participating providers. The PPO arranges for services to be provided, but does not provide the services. PPOs do not share economic risk. The PPO responds to requests for proposals (RFPs) from employers or other payers, including HMOs or business alliances. Patients often must choose from a list of network providers.

Primary Care Physician: The internist, pediatrician, ob-gyn, family practitioner, or the like, who often serves as the primary gatekeeper in the health care system. He or she is clinically and financially responsible for referral to specialists for additional services. Some HMOs and integrated health delivery systems are now placing psychologists in the primary care role.

Profiling: A system of evaluating network providers used by managed care firms as the basis for client referrals. Profiles reflect the usual pattern and length of treatment, location, practice structure, specialities, hours of availability, any complaints, and a history of the working relationship with the company's case managers.

Self-Funded/Self-Insured: A situation in which the employer takes all the responsibility for mental health and medical health care benefits payments. The employer often hires a third-party administrator to handle claims and payments.

Shared Risk: Payers and providers share the profits or losses under a capitated contract. The idea is that sharing risk will increase provider accountability and increase efficiency.

Subscriber: The person designated by the employer or insurance company as the primary person covered for services.

Third-Party Administrator: An insurance or risk management company that specializes in administering benefits plans.

Treatment Plan: The provider's proposal for treating a client based on diagnosis and clinical protocol and guidelines set by the managed care firm and agreed to by the provider. Case managers often work with the provider to amend treatment plans to fit benefit plans for covered clients. Treatment plans must be approved and followed in order for services to be reimbursed.

Utilization Management: A process of health care decision making that collects and analyzes information on diagnoses, treatment and service plans, costs, and statistical benchmarks for similar services. The goal is to determine the treatment that produces the best outcome for a diagnosis at the most efficient cost.

Utilization Review: The evaluation of the necessity, appropriateness, and efficiency of the use of behavioral health care services, procedures, and resources. Reviewed items include the treatment plan, intensity and level of care, treatment modality and setting, and medical/functional necessity.

Vertically Integrated System of Care: Sometimes referred to as an organized system of care, or a continuum of care. Currently held as a model for modern health care systems, this new system integrates the funding, self-insured employer, benefits manager/administrator, and providers in a coordinated, one-stop shopping system.

Withhold: A percentage of provider payment that is held as a set-aside until certain expense and profit levels are attained. If the standards are not met, then little or none of the withhold is paid out. Standards are usually based on the length, amount, and cost of services delivered. Withholds can be based on reduced fees for service as well as on capitation or at-risk arrangements.

APPENDIX B

PROVIDER GUIDELINES

MCC's *Level of Care Guidelines* is available to any provider. Write to S. Mahaffey, MHC and Associates, 1190 Portland Avenue S, Burnsville, MN 55337. The cost is $35 for a hardcover book, or $10 for a computer diskette. Clinical and provider guidelines are available over the Internet at MCC's home page (http://www.mcc-care.com).

Value Behavioral Health's *Provider Manual for Participating Providers* is free to all network providers when they sign contracts. Nonnetwork providers may purchase the manual for $50. Write to Value Behavioral Health, Corporate Provider Relations, 3110 Fairview Park Drive, Falls Church, VA 22042; 800-765-0903.

Comprehensive Behavioral Care, Inc., provides its *CBC Best Practice Guidelines* at no cost. Contact Provider Relations, CBC, 4200 West Cypress Street, Suite 300, Tampa, FL 33607; 813-872-1561, ext. 206.

CMG Health sells its *Best Practice Guidelines* for $25 to any provider. Send a check payable to CMG along with a letter requesting the guidelines to CMG Health, 25 Crossroads Drive, Owings Mills, MD 21117; 410-654-2645.

Merit Behavioral Care Corporation providers should receive a treatment guidelines and provider policy manual when signing contracts. The manuals are not available to nonnetwork providers. For a copy, network providers should call Merit Provider Relations at 800-999-9772, ext. 2992.

Green Spring Health Services policy and treatment guidelines are free to providers. They are not available to nonnetwork clinicians. Network providers may request a copy by calling Green Spring Provider Relations at 800-788-4005.

U.S. Behavioral Health provider guidelines are available to network providers only. The handbook will be automatically mailed to contracted providers. While USBH doesn't plan to sell its guidelines to nonnetwork providers, the company is willing to allow group practices to review the book before applying. Network providers who don't receive manuals should call USBH at 800-333-8724. *Note:* USBH is now merged with United Behavioral Systems at 9705 Data Park Drive, Minneapolis, MN 55440-1459; 800-551-7413.

APPENDIX C

MANAGED BEHAVIORAL HEALTH "CARVE-OUT" FIRMS

Although all network provider decisions were once handled through central offices of large national managed behavioral health care firms, there is now a trend toward regional network management. That's partly because of the companies' requirements to visit provider offices and inspect clinical records. Handling those reviews by regions is easier for the companies. In those cases, providers will be referred to the regional provider relations department for their locations.

ACORN Behavioral HealthCare Management Corporation.
134 North Narberth Avenue
Narberth, PA 19072-2299
800-223-7050

Anthem Health Inc.
4040 Vincennes Circle
Indianapolis, IN 46268
317-290-5743

Apogee
1018 West Ninth Avenue
King of Prussia, PA 19046
610-992-7670

Bradman/UniPsych Companies
7777 Davie Road Extension, Suite 302
Hollywood, FL 33024
954-704-8686

Ceridian Employer Services
8100 34th Avenue South
Minneapolis, MN 55425-1640
612-853-8100

CLM Behavioral Health Systems
44 Stiles Road
Salem, NH 03079
603-893-3548

CMG Health, Inc.
25 Crossroads Drive
Owings Mills, MD 21117
410-581-8800

CNR Health, Inc.
2400 South 102 Street, Suite 100
Milwaukee, WI 53227
414-327-5197

Comprehensive Behavioral Care
2203 North Lois Avenue, Suite 1205
Tampa, FL 33607
800-382-3259

ComPsych
455 North City Front Plaza, 24th Floor
Chicago, IL 60611
800-557-1005

CORPHEALTH
1300 Summit Avenue, Suite 600
Fort Worth, TX 76102
817-332-2519

Employee Assistance Associated, Inc.
900 Victors Way, Suite 350
Ann Arbor, MI 48108-2705
313-913-0606

Family Enterprises, Inc.
11700 West Lake Park Drive
Milwaukee, WI 53224
414-359-1055

First Mental Health
501 Great Circle Road, Suite 300
Nashville, TN 37228
615-256-3400

FPM Behavioral Health
1276 Minnesota Avenue
Winter Park, FL 32780
407-647-6153

Green Spring Health Services
The Clark Building, Suite 500
Columbia, MD 21044-2644
800-788-4005

Group Practice Affiliates
3414 Peachtree Drive NE
Atlanta, GA 30326
912-751-2270

Health Designs, Inc.
1201 South Alma School
Mesa, AZ 85210
800-600-5220

Health Management Strategies
1725 Duke Street, Suite 300
Alexandria, VA 22314
703-706-4100

Human Affairs International
P.O. Box 57986
Salt Lake City, UT 84157-0986
801-256-7000

Integra
1060 First Avenue, Suite 400
King of Prussia, PA 19406
610-992-7000

Integrated Behavioral Health
P.O. Box 30018
Laguna Nigel, CA 92607-0018
800-395-1616

MCC Behavioral Health
11095 Viking Drive, Suite 350
Eden Prairie, MN 55344
612-996-2000

MHN/OHS Foundation Health PsychCare Services, Inc.*
1600 Los Gamos Drive, Suite 300
San Rafael, CA 94903
800-541-3353
*Reflects the merger of Managed Health Network and OHS

Merit Behavioral Care Corporation
13736 Riverport Drive, Suite 444, 2nd Floor
Maryland Heights, MO 63043
800-999-9772

Mustard Seed
711 Valley Green Road, Suite 300
Fort Washington, PA 19034
215-233-9800

Northwestern Managed Mental Health Program
448 East Ontario, 8th Floor
Chicago, IL 60611
312-908-3910

Options Mental Health
240 Corporate Boulevard
Norfolk, VA 23502
757-459-5200

PacifiCare Behavioral Health, Inc.
23046 Avenida de la Carlota, Suite 700
Laguna Hills, CA 92653-5311
714-859-7971

PHC, Inc.
200 Lake Street, Suite 102
Peabody, MA 01960
508-536-2777

Plan 21
4550 Post Oak Place, Suite 341
Houston, TX 77027
800-622-7276 (Helen Dexter)

Perspectives Ltd.
111 North Wabash Avenue, Suite 1620
Chicago, IL 60602
800-456-6327

Principal Behavioral Health Care, Inc.
1801 Rockville Pike
Rockville, MD 20852
301-571-0633

PruPsych Management
24 Greenway Plaza, Suite 700
Houston, TX 77046
713-965-1000

Sheppard Pratt Health System, Inc.
6501 North Charles Street
Baltimore, MD 21285-6815
410-938-3150

The Holman Group
21050 Van Owen Street
Canoga Park, CA 91303
800-824-2932

United Behavioral Systems
9705 Data Park Drive
Minneapolis, MN 55343
612-945-6666

U.S. Behavioral Health
2000 Powell Street, Suite 1180
Emeryville, CA 94609
800-888-2998

U.S. Healthcare
9800 Jolly Road
Bluebell, PA 19422
800-323-9930

Value Behavioral Health
3110 Fairview Park Drive
Falls Church, VA 22042
703-205-7000

VISTA Health Plans
2355 Northside Drive
San Diego, CA 92108
800-303-5175

APPENDIX D

OUTCOMES MEASUREMENT TOOLS

Addiction Severity Index. DeltaMetrics, One Commerce Square, Suite 1020, 20005 Market Street, Philadelphia, PA 19103; 800-238-2433.

Basis-32. Behavioral and Symptom Identification Scale. Evaluative Service Unit, McLean Hospital, 115 Mill Street, Belmont, MA 02178-9106; 617-855-2425.

B.O.S.S. Beaumont Outcome Software System. Counseling Associates, Inc., 26699 West Twelve Mile Road, Suite 100, Southfield, MI 48034-7803; 810-353-5030.

GAF. Global Assessment of Functioning Scale. Found inside the DSM-IV manual available from the American Psychiatric Press. American Psychiatric Association, 1400 K Street, NW, Washington, DC 20005; 800-368-5777.

OQ-45.2. Outcome Questionnaire. Single page, 45 questions, copyrighted. American Professional Credentialing Services LLC, 10421 Stevenson Rd., Box 346, Stevenson, MD 21153-0346

SCL-90-R. Symptom Checklist. NCS Assessments, P.O. Box 1416, Minneapolis, MN 55440; 800-627-7271.

SF-36. A health status questionnaire, also available in 12-question format as SF-12. Medical Outcomes Trust, P.O. Box 1917, Boston, MA 02205-8516; 617-426-4046.

SUDDS. Substance Use Disorder Diagnosis Schedule. New Standards, Inc., 1080 Montreal Avenue, Suite 300, St. Paul, MN 55116; 612-690-1002.

Patient Satisfaction Tools

Many clinicians create their own satisfaction surveys to go with outcomes tools. Here are recommended tools.

CSQ-8. Client Satisfaction Questionnaire. Available from the Association for Ambulatory Behavioral Healthcare, 901 N. Washington Street, Suite 600, Alexandria, VA 23314; 703-836-2274.

MHCA Satisfaction System. Mental Health Corporations of America is a trade group of at least 120 entrepreneurial mental health centers that have developed their own satisfaction instrument. Participants can submit their data and get reports back on how their ratings compare with national norms. MHCA, 2846-A Remington Green Circle, Tallahassee, FL; 800-447-3068.

SSS-30. Service Satisfaction Scale. Assesses several factors of service including providers, manner, skill, perceived outcome, access and office procedures. Self-administered, or administered by office receptionist. Alcohol Research Group, Thomas Greenfield, 2000 Hearst Avenue, Suite 300, Berkeley, CA 94709; 510-642-5208.

For a more extensive listing of outcomes measurement tools, see *Behavioral Healthcare Outcomes: A Reference Guide to Measurement Tools,* available from the National Community Mental Healthcare Council, 12300 Twinbrook Parkway, Suite 320, Rockville, MD 20852; 301-984-6200. Non-member prepaid price is $27.

Source: Practice Strategies, Vol. 3(4), p. 8.

APPENDIX E

SAMPLE FORMS

Outpatient Utilization Review Authorization for Release of Information for Professional Review of Treatment

I, ______________________________ understand and agree that, in order
(name of person receiving service [please print])

to assure the quality of service provided me under my health plan, information regarding my personal history and that of my family, together with medical reports, reports of psychological tests which may have been administered, diagnosis and treatment plan reports, will be confidentially reviewed by my Provider(s) and the Behavioral Health Network. I understand that this review will be for the purpose of planning and evaluating the psychological services being made available to me through my health plan. The above-mentioned information may also be confidentially reviewed by a committee of Mental Health Professionals for quality assurance purposes and treatment outcome studies. Such a review would only be conducted in accordance with the strictest safeguards and standards of confidentiality.

I understand that appropriateness and effectiveness of treatment will be weighed in authorizing services.

I further understand that my treatment records are for the information only of persons who are professionally capable of understanding, appreciating, and acting upon them, using their specific and advanced professional training in the mental health field.

I hearby release the source of these records from any liability arising from their release. I authorize my Mental Health Professional to talk by telephone, by written material, or by facsimile about any aspect of my care that is necessary for effective treatment and in authorizing sessions.

A photocopy of this release is to be considered as valid as the original.

Date____/____/____Patient's Signature______________________________

Parent of Guardian's Signature______________________________

Source: Behavioral Health Network, Inc. Glendale, California.

Patient Information

You will be participating in a 1 to 12 session, brief, problem-oriented psychotherapeutic process. If at the end of therapy more supportive type treatment is needed, aftercare group therapy is available.

1) The issue of confidentiality needs to be clearly spelled out. You have the right to confidentiality and Mental Health Professionals are prohibited by law from revealing to any other person what you have said without your permission.

   However, there are limits to your rights under this law. In the following instances your right to confidentiality must be set aside and the law and professional ethics require that information disclosed be revealed even without your permission.

   a. If your mental condition becomes an issue in a lawsuit.
   b. Cases of sexual, physical, or severe emotional child or elder (anyone over 65 yrs.) abuse.
   c. If a person is a danger to herself/himself or others.
   d. Failure to assume financial responsibility for your bill might necessitate the use of collection procedures, which means providing them with limited privileged information.

2) It is expected that the copayment will be made at the conclusion of each session unless other arrangements have been made.
3) In the event that you must reschedule a session for whatever reason, it is important that your therapist be informed AT LEAST 48 HOURS IN ADVANCE. Without such notice, you agree to assume full financial responsibility, including your copay, for the professional time that was reserved for you. Your insurance company will not be billed for missed sessions.
4) This form serves as authorization for treatment of any minor children.
5) Since insurance billing is involved, this form authorizes the release of information to the insurance company via telephone, written, or facsimile transmission of treatment plans.
6) Sometimes, the psychotherapeutic process can bring up uncomfortable feelings and reactions, such as anxiety, sadness, anger, etc. Please be aware that this is a normal response to talking about unresolved life experiences and will be worked out between you and your therapist.
7) Individual session length will be determined by your therapist.

I HAVE READ AND UNDERSTAND THE INFORMATION IN THIS FORM.

____ ___/___/___

Signature of Patient (or Guardian) Date

Source: Behavioral Health Network, Inc. Glendale, California.

Patient Feedback

Dr. Blume & Associates

The success of our group practice depends upon your SATISFACTION with the services you received. Please take 5 minutes to tell us about your experience in our office. We are committed to quality treatment, delivered in a caring atmosphere and we need your feedback.

1. My therapist was ____________________. I was referred to Dr. Blume & Associates by ____ (name of person, agency, or relationship to you).

2. I participated in the following form(s) of therapy at Dr. Blume & Associates: Individual ( ) Couples ( ) Family ( ) Group ( ) A combination ( )

3. Approximate length of treatment at this office was ___ sessions / months / years (circle only one). My diagnosis was ____________________. Check here if you are not sure. ____

4. In addition to the above treatment, I also participated in additional treatment as described below:

   12-Step Program(s)____________ Self-Help Group(s)______________
   Diet Program ________________ Exercise Program ______________
   Medication (type)_____________ Day/Night Treatment ____________
   Other _______________________ Bibliotherapy (Readings) __________

5. Were you hospitalized during your course of treatment at our practice? Yes _____ No _____ If Yes, for how long (____ days) and where (_________ name of facility). If No, do you believe the quality of your outpatient treatment helped prevent hospitalization? Yes ___ No ___ N/A ___

6. Overall, I would rate the services received at Dr. Blume & Associates as (place an "**X**" on the line):

   Poor — Fair — Average — Good — Excellent

7. Have you had the experience with previous therapists with which you are comparing the therapy you received at Dr. Blume & Associates? Yes ___ No ___ N/A ___

8. I would ( ) would not ( ) refer other patients to this practice or return for additional treatment in the future. How could your therapist have been more helpful to you (or to your family)? What could we have done differently? ____

9. What was MOST HELPFUL in your treatment?_________________________

10. Were your presenting symptoms adequately addressed in the treatment? Yes___ No ___ How would you rate your overall improvement?

    Worse — No change — Some change — Significant positive change

11. Has your work performance improved during the course of or at the conclusion of your therapy in our office? Yes ___ No ___ N/A ___

12. Other comments you would like to make: ___________________________
    ____

Today's date: ____/____/____ *THANK YOU VERY MUCH FOR YOUR FEEDBACK*

CUSTOMER SATISFACTION SURVEY

Our service business depends on your complete satisfaction. Please take a few minutes to tell us how we are doing. Your helpful comments will guide us in reengineering the future of how we deliver services and conduct business.

THANK YOU,

Ginger Blume, Ph.D. & Associates

Place an "X" in the box that best describes your opinion on each of the items below. If an item is not relevant, place an "X" in the far-right column labeled "N/A."

	STRONGLY DISAGREE ↓	SOMEWHAT DISAGREE ↓	AGREE ↓	MOSTLY AGREE ↓	STRONGLY AGREE ↓	
WE PROMPTLY RETURN YOUR CALLS AND/OR RESPOND TO YOUR REQUESTS:						N/A —
CLIENTS ARE EASILY SCHEDULED FOR APPOINTMENTS WITH THIS OFFICE:						N/A —
OUR ADMINISTRATIVE STAFF IS PLEASANT AND HELPFUL:						N/A —
THERAPISTS PROVIDE RELEVANT AND HELPFUL CLINICAL FEEDBACK UPON REQUEST:						N/A —
OUR OFFICE IS CONVENIENTLY LOCATED, WITH ADEQUATE PARKING:						N/A —
CLIENTS APPEAR, OVERALL, TO BE PLEASED WITH OUR CLINICAL SERVICES:						N/A —

PLEASE FOLD TO MAIL

Source: Ginger Blum, Ph.D. & Associates, Middletown, CT. Used with permission.

BIBLIOGRAPHY

Note: Asterisks indicate the authors' top picks for the bookshelves of clinicians with limited time and budgets.

*Austad, C., & Berman, W. (Eds.) (1991). *Psychotherapy in managed health care: The optimal use of time and resources.* Washington, DC: American Psychological Association.

Baldor, R. (1996). *Managed care made simple.* Cambridge, MA: Blackwell.

Baxter, M. J., & Hornback, M. (1993). The evolution of medical staff credentialing. *Medical Staff Counselor,* Winter.

Berger, E. (1995). Specialty physician networks in managed care. *Health Care Innovations, 5*(July/Aug.), 16–18, 37–38.

*Boland, P. (Ed.) (1991). *Making managed health care work.* New York: McGraw-Hill.

*Browning, C., & Browning, B. (1993). *How to partner with managed care.* Los Alamitos, CA: Duncliff's International.

Buchanan, J., et al. (1992). *Cost and use of capitated medical services: Evaluation of the program for prepaid managed health care.* Santa Monica, CA: Rand.

Cagney, T., & Rush Woods, D. (1993). Provider selection in managed care. *Behavioral Healthcare Tomorrow, 2*(6), 38–39.

Cagney, T., & Rush Woods, D. (1994a). Clinical management information systems. *Behavioral Healthcare Tomorrow, 3*(1), 23–24.

Cagney, T., & Rush Woods, D. (1994b). Why focus on outcomes data? *Behavioral Healthcare Tomorrow, 3*(3), 23–24.

Corcoran, K., & Vandiver, V. (1996). *Maneuvering the maze of managed care: Skills for mental health practitioners.* New York: Free Press.

Daniels, A., & Freeman, M. (1994). The role of capitation in quality behavioral healthcare systems of the future. *Behavioral Healthcare Tomorrow, 3*(4), 79–80.

Danzi, T. (Ed.) (1996). *Positioning your practice for the managed care market.* Baltimore: Williams & Wilkins.

*Davis, J. (1995). *Marketing for therapists.* San Francisco: Jossey-Bass.

DeMuro, P. (1995). *The financial manager's guide to managed care and integrated delivery systems: Strategies for contracting compensation and reimbursement.* Burr Ridge, IL: Irwin.

DeMuro, R. (1994). *Integrated delivery systems.* Gaithersburg, MD: Aspen.

Emenhiser, D., DeWoodsy, M., & Barker, R. (1995). *Managed care: An agency guide to surviving and thriving.* Washington, DC: Child Welfare League of America.

Feldman, J., & Fitzpatrick, R. (Eds.) (1992). *Managed mental health care: Administrative and clinical issues.* Washington, DC: American Psychiatric Press.

Feldman, S. (Ed.) (1992). *Managed mental health services.* Springfield, IL: C C Thomas.

Feldman, S., & Goldman, W. (Eds.) (1993). *Managed mental health care.* San Francisco: Jossey-Bass.

Freeman, M., & Trabin, T. (1994, Oct.). *Managed behavioral healthcare: History, models, key issues, and future course.* White Paper for the U.S. Center for Mental Health Services.

Gardner, J. M. (1994). Implementation of a provider credentialing/recredentialing process and development of a physician profile in an IPO-model HMO. *Medical Interface, 7*(8), 102–105, 108, 117.

Garfield, W., & Bergin, A. (1986). *Handbook of psychotherapy and behavior change* (3rd. ed.) New York: Wiley.

Garfield, S. L., & Bergin, A. E. (Eds.). (1994). *Handbook of psychotherapy and behavior change* (4th ed.). New York: Wiley.

Giles, T. (1993). *Managed mental health care: A guide for practitioners, employers and hospital administrators.* Boston: Allyn & Bacon.

Goodman, M., Brown, J., & Deitz, P. (1992). *Managing managed care: A mental health practitioner's survival guide.* Washington, DC: American Psychiatric Press.

Grant, P., & Smith, P. (1992). *Legal issues related to the formation and restructuring of integrated medical groups and new models in hospital-medical group affiliation.* San Francisco: Davis Wright Tremaine.

Greenberg, D. (1996). Gloomy new year for US health industry. *Lancet, 347,* 51.

Hale, J. A., & Hunter, M. M. (1988). *From HMO movement to managed care industry: The future of HMOs in a volatile healthcare market.* Excelsior, MN: Center for Managed Care Research.

Harris, S. (1991, Dec.). Treatment planning: A managed care guide to rules of the road. *California Psychological Association Briefings: Managed Care,* no. 107.

Hoyt, M. (1995). *Brief therapy and managed care: Readings for contemporary practice.* San Francisco: Jossey-Bass.

Hymowitz, C. (1995, Dec. 21). High anxiety, in the name of Freud, why are psychiatrists complaining so much? The new economics of mental health. *Wall Street Journal,* p. A1.

Jackson, V., Geraty, R., & Marques, C. (1993). Are we training too many mental health providers? *Behavioral Healthcare Tomorrow, 2*(6), 26–28.

Johnson, L. (1995). *Psychotherapy in the age of accountability.* New York: Norton.

Joint Commission on Accreditation of Healthcare Organizations (1989). *Managed care standards manual.* Chicago: Author.

Kaluzny, A., Zuckerman, H., & Ricketts, R. (Eds.) (1995). *Partners for the dance: Forming strategic alliances in health care.* Ann Arbor, MI: Health Administration Press.

Kongsveldt, P. (Ed.) (1995). *Essentials of managed care.* Gaithersburg, MD: Aspen.

Lambert, M. J., & Bergin, W. E. (1994). The effectiveness of psychotherapy. In S. Garfield & A. Bergin (Eds.), *Handbook of psychotherapy and behavior change* (4th ed.). New York: Wiley.

Lee, D. (1995). *Capitation: The physician's guide.* Chicago: American Medical Association.

MacKenzie, R. (1995). *Effective use of group therapy in managed care.* Washington, DC: American Psychiatric Press.

Merli, G., et al. (1996). *Managed care and office practice.* Philadelphia: Saunders.

Patient experiences with managed care: A survey (1995). New York: Commonwealth Fund.

Polonsky, I. (1995). How to write treatment reports for managed care. *California Therapist, 7*(1).

*Poynter, W. (1994). *The preferred provider's handbook: Building a successful private therapy practice in the managed care marketplace.* New York: Brunner/Mazel.

Pyenson, B. (Ed.) (1995). *Calculated risk: A provider's guide to assessing and controlling the financial risk of managed care.* Chicago: American Hospital Publishing.

Redick, R., Witkin, M., Atay, J., & Manderscheid, R. (1994, May). Expansion of mental health care in the United States between 1955 and 1990. *Mental Health Statistical Note 210,* U.S. Department of Health and Human Services, Center for Mental Health Services.

Ruben, D., & Stout, C. (1993). *Transitions: Handbook of managed care for inpatient to outpatient treatment.* Westport, CT: Prager.

Sabin, J., & Daniels, N. (1994). Determining "medical necessity" in mental health practice. *Hastings Center Report,* no. 6.

Samuels, D. (1996). *Capitation: New opportunities in healthcare delivery.* Chicago: Irwin.

Schereger, J. (1993). *Successful practice management in the age of managed care* (video). Secaucus, NJ: Network for Continuing Medical Education.

Schreter, R., Sharfstein, C., & Sharfstein, S. (Eds.) (1994). *Allies and adversaries: The impact of managed care on mental health services.* Washington, DC: American Psychiatric Press.

Shenson, H. (1990). *The contract and fee-setting guide for consultants and professionals.* New York: Wiley.

Shroyer, S. (1996, Jan./Feb.). Using electronic credentialing to address the quality revolution. *Infocare* pp. 40–42.

Sollins, H. L. (1995). *Hold that pen: Answers to your contracting questions.* Presentation to the American Association for Marriage and Family Therapy, Baltimore.

Sperry, L. (1995). *Psychopharmacology and psychotherapy: Strategies for maximizing treatment outcomes.* New York: Brunner/Mazel.

Talmon, M. (1990). *Single session intervention.* San Francisco: Jossey-Bass.

Theis, G. (1992). Behavioral health care services: Emerging concepts. *AAPPO Journal, 2*(6), 9–12.

Tuttle, G. (1996). Less paperwork? Large MCOs promise standard forms and one provider application this year. *Practice Strategies, 2*(1), 1–2.

*Winegar, N. (1992). *The clinician's guide to managed mental health care.* New York: Haworth.

Winston, A. (Ed.) (1985). *Clinical and research issues in short-term dynamic psycotherapy.* Washington, DC: American Psychiatric Press.

Woolley, S. (1993, Sept. 13). Physician, restrain thyself. *Business Week,* pp. 32–33.

Youngberg, B. (Ed.) (1996). *Managing the risks of managed care.* Gaithersburg, MD: Aspen.

*Zieman, G. (1995). *The complete capitation handbook: How to design and implement at-risk contracts for behavioral healthcare.* San Francisco: Jossey-Bass.

INDEX